LEMON & LIME
LIBRARY

LEMON & LIME LIBRARY
An articulation screen & resource pack

Rebecca Palmer & Athanassios Protopapas

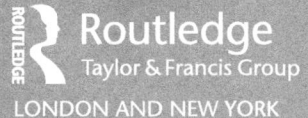

Routledge
Taylor & Francis Group

LONDON AND NEW YORK

First published 2008 by Speechmark Publishing Ltd.

Published 2017 by Routledge
2 Park Square, Milton Park, Abingdon, Oxon OX14 4RN
711 Third Avenue, New York, NY 10017, USA

Routledge is an imprint of the Taylor & Francis Group, an informa business

British Library Cataloguing in Publication Data
Palmer, Rebecca
    Lemon and lime library: an articulation resource pack
    1. Communicative disorders – Diagnosis 2. Communicative disorders – Treatment
    I. Title II. Protopapas, Athanassios
    616.8'55

ISBN-13: 9780863885488 (pbk)

CONTENTS

LIST OF FIGURES & TABLES

Figures

Tables

PREFACE

THE LEMON & LIME LIBRARY provides a wealth of material for use with clients with articulation disorders, including an articulation screening test, words systematically selected according to linguistic and phonetic criteria, and fun sentences and tongue twisters. The material can be found in the book or can be accessed quickly from a CD database by filling in the required phonetic criteria on a colourful and simple screen. The same screen allows you to design worksheets with words, pictures and instructions for each individual. The versatile resource will be invaluable to speech & language therapists, teachers and students beginning to get to grips with phonetics!

ACKNOWLEDGEMENTS

DEVELOPMENT OF THIS BOOK and accompanying CD-Rom was supported in part by the European Commission contract QLG5-CT-2001-01971 for the research and technological development project 'Ortho-Logo-Paedia' (OLP) in the context of 'Quality of Life and Management of Living Resources' of the 5th Framework Programme.

The software in the accompanying CD-Rom was developed at the Institute for Language & Speech Processing by engineers Evagelia Tsiligianni (python interface) and Giannis Koulafetis (MS Access library).

PART I

INTRODUCTION

What is the Lemon & Lime Library?

The Lemon & Lime Library is a resource pack for speech & language therapists that provides a wealth of written and picture material to be used in the screening and treatment of articulation disorders. This resource is intended: (1) to help therapists profile the articulation ability of a client; (2) to identify areas in particular need of treatment; (3) to provide the material and tools to create tailor-made practice worksheets. Word lists have been systematically produced so that words containing sounds in different positions and in different lengths of word and phrase can be easily found. All words selected have a frequency of more than ten per million (according to the British National Corpus) to keep word frequency as a constant variable in articulation practice (Leech *et al*, 2001). An accompanying CD-Rom holds a database of the Lemon & Lime Library from which words can be selected to create worksheets tailor-made to the individual client.

Who is the Lemon & Lime Library useful for?

The material in the resource pack is suitable for use with clients of all ages. The resource is flexible and therapists can add familiar words or remove unfamiliar words, as appropriate. The material can be presented to clients in words or pictures, making it widely accessible.

The pack was designed to provide a resource for speech & language therapists who are working with articulation disorders; but the material may also be of benefit to teachers and to speech therapy students. In order to generate words with specific criteria, users need to be familiar with the phonetic labels as the library is organised by phonetic class and by length of phonetic unit. The CD-Rom can help students become adept at using phonetic labels by providing feedback in the form of word lists once the phonetic criteria have been filled in. If the incorrect words do not appear there is no harm done! Just think about which label may have been incorrect and change it until you see the words you intended. Not only phonetic, but also linguistic properties such as word imageability are defined for all words in the Lemon & Lime Library. As such, it may also be a useful resource for linguistic research purposes.

What does the Lemon & Lime Library contain?

The resource pack is divided into three parts: the articulation screening test; the resource library and the library of phrases and sentences.

1 *Articulation screening test*

The screening test contains 96 words, which between them contain examples of all the English phonemes in all different word positions. A phonemic or phonetic transcription of these words can contribute to producing a profile of a client's articulation patterns. Alternatively, a phoneme distortion scale has been devised for use in cases where phonetic transcription may be complex. For example, in dysarthria articulation errors are distortions of the target phoneme that require a narrow phonetic transcription, rather than substitutions with other discrete phonemes for which a broad transcription will usually suffice. The screen provides a useful baseline of articulation and highlights areas in need of treatment. The words selected for the screening test do not duplicate any of the words that appear in the treatment lists, and therefore truly assess generalisation of sounds at word level.

2 *Resource library for treatment of sounds and words*

Lists of sounds and words available for practice are organised into levels according to the length of the linguistic unit. Table 2.1 on page 11 lists the seven levels of practice, level 1 being the simplest level. Word lists for each level are available in this book and can be photocopied for use with clients. They are also available on CD-Rom.

3 *Library of phrases and sentences*

The final part of the package contains fun phrases and sentences organised according to the sounds they target. There are short phrases containing only one word with the target sound and phrases and sentences of increasing length that either include several examples of one target sound eg voiceless bilabial plosive /p/, or examples of a range of sounds made in a particular place eg bilabials /p/, /b/ and /m/. These phrases and sentences can be photocopied from the booklet for use with clients.

The Lemon & Lime Library on CD-Rom

What the CD-Rom provides

1 Instead of searching for words in the book the user can type in the phonetic criteria required, filling in each field with help from drop-down menus. Criteria include:

- place and manner of articulation
- voicing
- position of the sound in a word
- level of practice
- number of syllables
- imageability
- clusters

If the user does not mind about a certain criterion, the field can be left blank. For example, if you require bilabial stops but do not have a preference for voiced or voiceless stops, leaving the field blank will result in presentation of both. When any criteria have been filled in, the computer automatically generates the list of words.

2 Words can be selected for a specific client. For example, if a word produced in the list may not be understood, or has unwanted associations for the client, it need not be selected.

3 Additionally, words can be added that are important to an individual client but are not currently in the database. The phonetic criteria matching this word need to be filled in and then this word will appear in the client's list. It will also be saved in the database. In this way, the database of words can be built up over time and can store a large number of words.

4 A worksheet can then be designed for an individual client with the option to add pictures representing imageable words for clients who cannot read. All worksheets can be printed out for distribution to clients.

5 Pictures can be added by selecting words that are imageable and checking the box labelled 'print pictures' at the bottom right of the lemon side of the screen.

How to use the Lemon & Lime Library on CD-Rom

This software runs on PCs only and is compatible with Windows 2000, XP and Vista. It requires a minimum screen resolution of 1024 × 768. This program must first be installed on your computer in order to run. The CD-Rom must then always be inserted in your CD-Rom drive every time you want to run the program.

To install the program on your computer

1   Insert the CD-Rom into your machine.

2   It should autostart.

3   If the installer program does not start automatically follow these instructions:
    - Double-click on 'My Computer' *then either*:
        - Double-click on the Lemon & Lime icon.
        - *Or* right-click on the CD drive or the Lemon & Lime icon displayed on the screen and select 'Open' or 'Explore' in the pop-up menu.
    - *Then* double-click on Setup.exe and follow the prompts.

4   When prompted by the installer program, click on 'Next' until finished. Installation proceeds automatically. Once installed, the program can be opened from the Programs list under 'Start'.

When opened, the program presents the Lemon & Lime screen as shown in Figure 1.1. Criteria can be specified in the Lime (left-hand) section and available items that satisfy your criteria will appear as a list. The personalised list can be constructed in the Lemon (right-hand) section and any notes and information added. This can then be printed out.

Selecting from available items

To select from items already available in the library, select 'Search in library' at the top of the Lime-coloured section. Use as many of the listed selection criteria as you like. Each criterion has a drop-down menu. When you click on the empty field, a list of

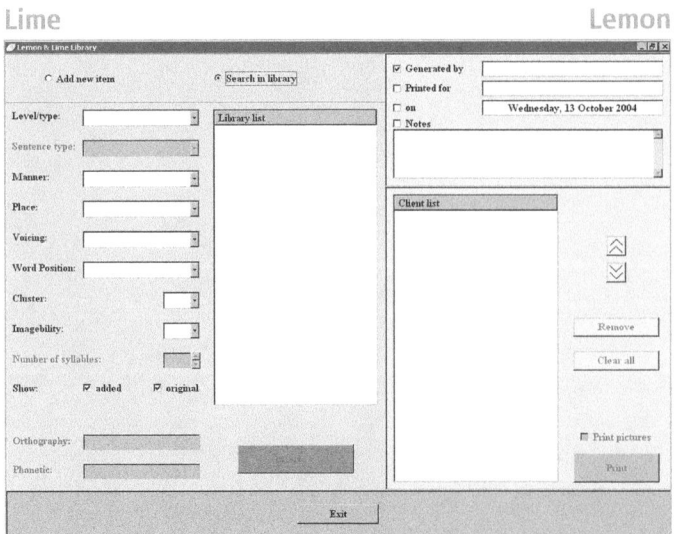

FIGURE 1.1

Starting screen of Lemon & Lime Library program

available choices appears, and you can make your selection. As soon as you have selected at least one criterion, all available items in the library will appear in the 'Library list' space. By selecting more criteria, the list is further restricted.

To remove a single criterion and prevent it from affecting your word list, right-click on this particular criterion and a 'Cut/Copy/Paste/Delete' menu will appear. Click on 'Delete' to reset the criterion.

To create personalised worksheets, by adding your name, the client's name, or the date you want the worksheet to be used (today's date will automatically appear) and any other instructions and notes for the client, fill in the boxes at the top of the Lemon section and click on the corresponding check boxes. Remember that only fields with a check mark will appear on the printout.

To create the client list select any items from the Library list, click on them (this automatically highlights them) and then click 'Insert'. This will transfer the items to the client list in the Lemon section. You can click on individual items and 'Insert', shift and click to select successive items or control and click to add an individual item to your selection. To select *all* of the listed items, right-click in the list area and then click on 'Select all'. You can repeat selection and insertion as many times as you like.

Using imageable words. Imageability is one of the selection criteria in the Lime section. If a word is imageable, an image icon (🖐) will appear next to the word once it is in the client list area. Click on the 'print pictures' check box to ensure that the picture is printed.

To add an item not available in the library, select 'Add new item' at the top of the Lime section. Type your word in the 'Orthography' box. Select the relevant criteria for your word, otherwise you will not be able to find it later based on its phonetic properties. When done, click on 'Insert' to add this new item both to your client list on the Lemon side and to the program Library for future use. When searching for items in the library, you can choose to view original and/or your added items by checking the 'added' or 'original' boxes next to 'Show' in the Lime section. Items you have added will always appear in the list with a red bullet point (●) next to them.

To change the order of items in your client list on the Lemon section, select an item you wish to move and click on the double up/down arrow (⩓ ⩔).

To remove an item from the client list, click on it to highlight it and then click on 'Remove'.

To print your client's list along with any notes and other information, click 'Print' at the bottom right-hand side of the Lemon section. If you have selected only imageable items, you may choose to print the corresponding pictures by clicking the 'Print pictures' box before printing.

To clear your list and start afresh, click on 'Clear all' and confirm your intention in the window that will appear.

Two approaches to the treatment of articulation are often described. The first is commonly described as the **traditional approach**, which focuses on sounds sufficiently deviant from a normative standard (Fletcher, 1992). In this approach, the basic articulatory skills are achieved through speech sound drills (repeating the sound over and over) before combining the target sound with vowels then consonant-vowel-consonant combinations and so on, gradually expanding the context in which sounds are presented.

The second approach is known as a **cognitive-linguistic** or **phonological approach**, which is based on the assumption that 'articulation errors are evidence of a phonological disorder' (Fletcher, 1992). This approach therefore views articulation disturbances as reflections of rule-based errors rather than motor deficiencies, and works on classes of sounds with common phonetic features in remediation.

The above description of the treatment approaches suggests that there are traditional and new methods of treating disorders of speech sound production. 'Articulation' has been used as an umbrella term for speech sound production. However, if we define 'articulation' still further it becomes clear that the two approaches mentioned above are not 'traditional' and 'new' so much as different strategies for treating speech production where errors are due to disorders at different levels of the speech production process.

Figure 2.1 offers a suggestion for the hierarchy of the levels at which speech production can break down, closely based on currently accepted models of language processing (Kay *et al*, 1992; Yorkston *et al*, 1999). At the level of cognition an idea is formed that the speaker wishes to express. Errors at this level may be caused by dementia or dysphasia. Once the idea is formed, language skills are used to select sentence structures and words to convey the intended meaning. This level may also be disrupted by dysphasia or language learning delays and disorders. Next, the sounds required by the selected words are retrieved. Although this process relates to the sounds that are spoken, it can also be considered part of language as it is still controlled by the language centres of the brain. Errors due to delayed development of speech sound classes or disorders of the organisation of speech sounds, commonly referred to as phonological delays and disorders, have their origins at this level. Articulation is defined as follows by Yorkston *et al*.

> *Articulation is considered to be the movement of speech structures employed in the sounds of speech.* (Yorkston *et al*, 1999, p440)

If this is the case then we can reserve the use of the term 'articulation' for the lowest two boxes of the model: motor planning, where physical gestures are matched to the speech sounds; motor production, where the anatomy and physiology of speech work together to produce the sounds of speech. Dyspraxia or apraxia of speech is a disorder of motor planning. Motor production disorders may be isolated difficulties such as use of an interdental or lateral /s/, a result of a structural problem such as cleft lip and or palate, or a result of neurological impairment including the dysarthrias.

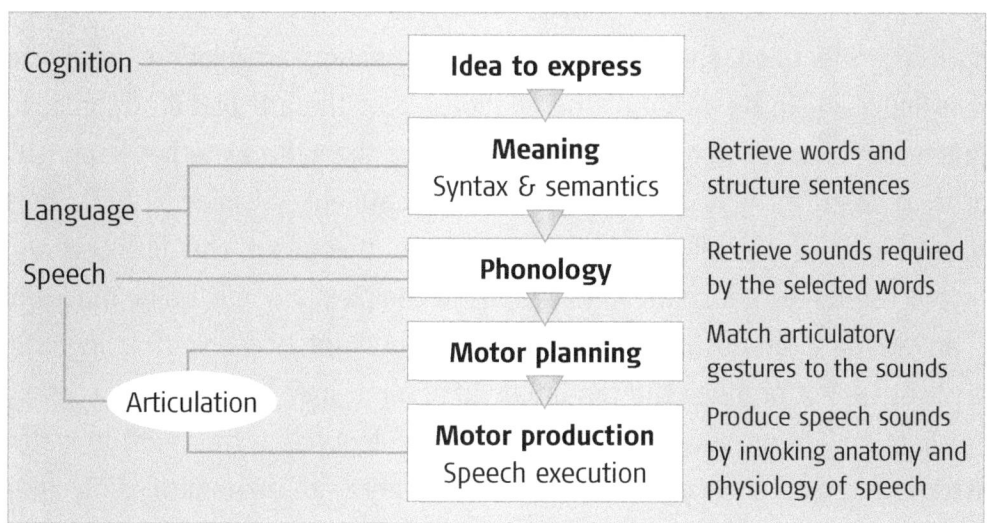

FIGURE 1.2 *A model of speech production*

Phonological-based treatment

The cognitive linguistic or phonological approach is appropriate for clients with speech disorders originating from above the level of articulation where he or she has usually not learned to use sound classes contrastively. Phonological based treatment should therefore first identify which phonological processes are at work and causing the errors and then begin work on a target sound class rather than single sound. For example, a common process is 'fronting' where velar plosives /k/ and /g/ are replaced by alveolar plosives /t/ and /d/. The cognitive-linguistic approach would always use words beginning with /k/ and /t/ in therapy, gradually encouraging the speaker to identify the differences and use the sounds contrastively. For example, minimal pairs such as 'key' and 'tea' may first be used to get the speaker to hear the difference, and then to encourage the words to be produced differently. Work usually begins with small units, eg the syllable, and builds up to words of greater length, then phrases and so on. There are many books which detail such phonology treatment such as *Clinical phonology* (Grunwell, 1992) and the *Metaphon Resource Pack* (Dean *et al*, 1991). As well as Howell & Dean (1991) and Kay *et al* (1992).

Treatment of speech sound disorders at articulation level

Speech sound disorders that arise at the level of articulation are motor speech disorders and as such treatment targets motor speech skills. Such a treatment is akin to the traditional articulation approach in that sounds particularly difficult to make or deviating from the norm are identified and remediated. When treating articulation deficits in dysarthria it is important to be aware of the relationship of the articulation disorder to deficits in other physiological systems; eg if movement of the soft palate has improved, nasal versus oral contrasts may be appropriate for treatment (Swigert, 1997). It is common to start with the smallest phonetic structure the client can produce and progressively practise the target sound in longer, more complex phonetic units, gradually introducing an accurate production of the target sound into meaningful linguistic context. If a client cannot produce the target sound at all, it may be helpful to start by teaching the client how to produce the sound in isolation by getting the client to watch the therapist and listen to an accurate sound. Where there are anatomical difficulties such as muscle weakness or altered structure of the articulators, it may be most helpful to focus on the speech end product, encouraging the client to alter articulation to get the sound closer to an accurate model rather than instructing the client where to place his or her articulators. Such modification based on speech end product is recommended by Yorkston *et al* (1999), who also describe contrastive production drills. This is where the client is encouraged to make two sounds that they produce in a similar way to sound as different as possible. Where the speech disorder is severe, this can help increase the range of sounds produced, thus enabling the client to make a greater distinction between words with different meanings (Yorkston *et al*, 1999). Swigert recommends drilling of lists of words that are being practised and using intelligibility as feedback to the client. In this type of activity, the client picks a word and says it; the therapist identifies which word she heard indicating to the client when the word needs to be produced more distinctively to relate the intended meaning (Swigert, 1997).

The Lemon & Lime Library is organised by phonetic class and by length of phonetic unit. Although initially designed for use with disorders of articulation (hence the title), words can be selected and worksheets designed also for use with clients with phonological speech disorders or word retrieval difficulties.

Criteria for the selection of words

The word library was initially developed to be used in conjunction with speech recognition technology tools in a computer program. The program required a means of selecting words that a client might need to practise so a library of words was produced, using strict criteria for their selection. Table 2.1 summarises the criteria used.

TABLE 2.1 *Criteria for words used to create a library*

1	All words chosen are real words used in British English speech. All words were therefore selected from the British National Corpus.
2	The library should be comprehensive. Therefore, all English phonemes are presented in all word positions, except those that do not occur in English, or occur in less than ten per million words.
3	Presentation of each consonant cluster possible in English in word initial position.
4	Presentation of multisyllabic words to look at effect of word length on articulation ability/intelligibility. A variety of stress placements was used to account for different rhythms/change in rhythm.
5	The British National Corpus contains 757,087 word forms, over half of which (52.44%) occur only once. All words chosen have a frequency of more than ten per million and are therefore high frequency words. This is to help limit potential effects of ease of word retrieval on production/articulation of the target word.
6	Variety of back, front, high, low, spread, round, long, short, diphthong, monophthong vowels used following and preceding each phonemic group to account for effects of different vowels on the production of consonants, and to assess vowel distortions if present.

How the library material is organised

Levels of articulation

The words have been organised so that they can be easily and logically accessed for use in therapy. 'Levels' have been allocated to articulation therapy as a way of organising the words. The levels correspond to the progression from practising isolated phonemes of difficulty (level 1) to combining them with vowels, practising them in different word positions, and then increasing the length of word until the client is able to practise using the target sound in the connected speech of phrases and sentences. The levels are shown in Table 2.2.

TABLE 2.2 *Levels of articulation therapy*

Level of practice	Linguistic unit
LEVEL 1	Single sounds
LEVEL 2	Consonant vowel/vowel consonant syllables
LEVEL 3	DDK rates – repetition of the same syllable
LEVEL 4	DDK rates – alternation of different syllables
LEVEL 5	Short words (two syllables)
LEVEL 6	Multisyllabic words
LEVEL 7	Phrases and sentences

Within each level, the words are organised to reflect where the target sound appears: in word initial, medial or final position.

Phrases and sentences (Level 7)

Phrases and sentences are often used in speech therapy when the client has mastered the target sound in isolation and in different word positions. They have been developed to reflect the lengthening of linguistic units used in articulation practice.

The phrase or sentence is organised according to the target phoneme. For each phoneme, the first set of Level 7 material contains short phrases and sentences with the target sound represented in only one word. Lists are further divided into whether the target phoneme appears before a short or long vowel, or a diphthong. Phrases and sentences then increase in length in the second set and contain several words with the target phoneme.

Motor learning theory suggests that after drilling desired behaviours separately, varying the behaviours practised is beneficial to their generalisation to spontaneous use (Wulf & Schmidt, 1997; Palmer & Meyer, 2000). With this in mind, tongue twisters have been developed containing different sounds made at the same place of articulation, that is, varying in manner or voicing.

How to retrieve words from the library database

In order to build an electronic database of the library, each sound and word has been given a code to identify its level and its phonetic features. This means that the correct words are retrieved from the database when the phonetic criteria fields are filled in by the clinician (see below).

How to create a personalised worksheet

The strength of creating a worksheet electronically is that it looks professional and personal at the same time.

1   We suggest that useful heading information needs to include the name of the client for which the worksheet is being specifically made, the date on which it is created and who is creating it. As individual clients respond to different explanations of how to achieve a particular articulatory target, a field for this very individual specific information has been created ('Notes').

2   As some clients cannot read or prefer the more stimulating presentation of a word in picture form, an option to put pictures on the worksheet has been included.

3   Most importantly a hard copy of the practice worksheet can be printed off and given to the client.

Phonetic selection criteria

1   The clinician needs to select the phonetic criteria of *place*, *manner* and *voicing*. Lists of phonetic labels for possible phonetic places and manners, and voiced/unvoiced have been organised so they can be selected from drop-down menus.

2   The position in which the phoneme is presented, eg word initial, word medial or word final, is important in the selection of words for articulation therapy. These options are given in a drop-down menu.

3   An additional phonetic consideration was the presentation of the chosen phoneme in consonant clusters or single consonants. All English consonant clusters are represented in words in the library so that consonants can be practised in clusters if the 'consonant' option is selected.

4   The level of articulation therapy can also be selected. Each level appears in a drop-down menu associated with the 'level' field.

5   The imageability of the word is thought to be an important criterion upon which to select words, particularly if picture material is required for the client. Illustrations have been made available for each word presented when the 'imageable' criterion is

selected. To print out pictures of the imageable words, check 'print pictures' on the lemon side of the CD-Rom screen.

6   The number of syllables in multisyllabic words is also considered a possible criterion on which to restrict the selection.

Amend the list of words to suit the client

1   If the list of words retrieved from the database is suitable for the intended client, it is possible to simply 'Select all' (when the right mouse button is clicked over the word list area).

2   If the list of words retrieved from the database containing the phonetic criteria selected is too large for a client to practise, then you can select just a few of the words by highlighting only those words required from the list presented on the lime side and then clicking 'insert' to transfer them to the 'lemon' section for printing on the worksheet.

3   There may be words containing the target sound in the client's environment that do not appear in the database: for example, the name of a pet. Words can be added to the list of the client's practise words by selecting 'add new item' at the top left of the lime section of the screen, typing the word into the box labelled 'orthography' (bottom left of lime section), and then clicking 'insert' to transfer the new word to the lemon side for printing on the client's worksheet. They are also stored in the database under the relevant phonetic criteria for future use if these criteria are selected once the word has been written in the 'orthography' box.

Articulation screening test – how it works

This screening test containing 96 words has been developed to assist therapists in identifying the phonemes in particular need of remediation. Each phoneme is sampled at least once in each word position. The screen also tests consonant clusters and multisyllabic words with a variety of stress patterns. The words have all been selected from the British National Corpus (Leech *et al*, 2001) using the same criteria as for the words selected for the library (see Table 2.1). **None of the words in the test are included in the library database so that the test can be re-administered following therapy** to see if articulation of a target phoneme has generalised to nontreated words. To make the screening test useful to as wide a range of clients as possible, it offers a choice of written words or pictures.

The words produced by the client during the test can be phonemically or phonetically transcribed. In addition, a distortion scale has been developed to indicate the severity of the articulation of each phoneme based on the perception of the therapist. This scoring system was developed for use by therapists, particularly in the analysis of speech that includes distorted target phonemes rather than those substituted with an incorrect English phoneme. Yorkston *et al* (1999) noted that articulation inventories are not in widespread clinical use for dysarthria. They propose that this may be due to the fact that 'distortions rather than substitutions or omissions predominate' which requires a narrow phonetic transcription. This is time consuming and the clinician cannot necessarily identify correctly what is going on inside the client's mouth to cause the distorted sound, thus reducing the reliability of the transcription. Additionally, Ball *et al* (1996) note that a phonetic transcription does not provide the clinician with a measure of severity.

The scoring system developed in this articulation resource attempts to enable analysis of distorted speech in an efficient and systematic way, being less time consuming than an accurate narrow phonetic transcription. Although not as informative as a phonetic transcription, the use of a distortion scale was felt to be an appropriate tool to use with a screening test, whose nature is to provide a first indication of particularly problematic phonemes relatively quickly. The scores can also be summed to indicate the severity of the disorder.

To further assist therapists with rapid identification of where articulation is particularly difficult, an analysis chart has been developed whereby scores for each sound in each position are summed and the total score is allocated to the correct box on the analysis chart. Areas displaying high scores therefore indicate the areas of most difficulty. Some sounds may be represented more frequently in the articulation screen, making the total error score for that sound more likely to be amongst the highest. This is acceptable, as sounds occurring frequently in the screen also occur frequently in speech. Therefore a high score for these sounds represents a greater impact on speech than that of a less frequently used sound.

Reliability of the distortion scale

In a pilot study conducted as part of the Ortho-Logo-Paedia project, the articulation screening test was carried out with a 43-year-old woman with mild-moderate ataxic dysarthria. Her reading of the 96 screening test words was recorded on minidisk and later played to seven speech & language therapists. Although the absolute scores totalled for each phoneme in each word position differed slightly between therapists, the highest scores allocated were for /s/ and /z/ for everyone. This resulting articulation profile led six of the seven therapists to identify word initial /s/ as a target for therapy. As a screening tool consistently directing therapists towards a common therapy objective, the distortion scale can be said to be reliable.

PART II

Articulation screening test

3 ARTICULATION SCREENING TEST

Instructions for use

This test is a screen to assist therapists in producing a profile of a client's articulation ability to help identify areas that might benefit from treatment. It is not standardised and as such there are no prescriptive instructions for use, so the test can be used at the therapist's discretion to assist in decision making and evaluating therapy. However, after using the test extensively during the trial of the Ortho-Logo-Paedia therapy programme with speakers with dysarthria, the authors' recommendations may be useful.

1   If you suspect many articulation errors, it may be difficult and less accurate to score online. For speakers with moderate to severe dysarthria, recording the production of the words and playing them back later to be scored can be beneficial. When the disorder is mild, it is possible to score online without difficulty once the clinician is familiar with the scoring system.

2   A phonemic transcription of words is sufficient if errors are mainly phoneme substitutions. Where a narrow transcription is required, the exact nature of the error may be difficult to identify or too time consuming. In this situation you may find it sufficient to use the distortion scale provided in order to quickly identify areas to target in therapy. Once the target phonemes have been identified, the words containing those phonemes could be analysed in more detail using a narrow phonetic transcription.

3   The screening material is provided in this book. On one side of the page written words are presented and on the reverse side the corresponding picture is shown. The use of the picture version of the screen is useful if the client cannot read. In addition, you may wish to consider that naming pictures may give a more spontaneous production of the target phonemes than reading written words.

Scoring instructions

All words on the scoring sheet are written orthographically and the received pronunciation (RP) of each word has been transcribed using the English phonemes defined by Gimson (1980):

1 Circle the sound in the word that you perceive to be distorted.

2 In the space next to the word indicate the level of distortion. Use the following codes:
   - a mild distortion: 1
   - a moderate distortion: 2
   - a severely distorted sound: 3
   - sound substituted with a totally different phoneme: 4
   - sound omitted altogether: 5

These scores are printed on the scoring sheet as a reminder. If more than one sound in the same word is distorted, circle them in order and write the distortion scores in the respective order.

Instructions for analysis

Find all of the words in which you circled phonemes. It is recommended that you add up the scores for /p/ then /b/, /m/ and so on, working your way systematically along the analysis chart for consonants and then for vowels. A pattern should begin to emerge with some sounds having much higher total scores than others. You may wish to highlight these, as you are likely to want to consider those sounds as targets for articulation therapy. The chart also provides space for you to make notes on additional observations or on the reasons for selecting particular phonemes for therapy. The scoring and analysis sheets on pages 20–22 can be photocopied for use with clients.

ARTICULATION SCREENING TEST

Scoring sheet and analysis charts

Scoring system Circle the part of the word that is distorted and add the distortion score to the adjacent box. The written word presentation of the test is presented first, followed by illustrations for the picture naming presentation of the test. The words in **bold** are illustrated.

①	mild distortion
②	moderate distortion
③	severe distortion
④	substitution with a different English phoneme
⑤	phoneme omitted from the word

Word		Score	Word		Score	Word		Score
1 **pen**	/pen/		21 **feet**	/fiːt/		41 red	/red/	
2 hoping	/həupɪŋ/		22 **fish**	/fɪʃ/		42 **nose**	/nəʊz/	
3 **cap**	/kæp/		23 **fourth**	/fɔːθ/		43 looking	/lʊkɪŋ/	
4 tip	/tɪp/		24 **laughing**	/læfɪŋ/		44 younger	/jʌŋgə/	
5 **paper**	/peɪpə/		25 **lorry**	/lɒrɪ/		45 zone	/zəʊn/	
6 **bag**	/bæg/		26 **van**	/væn/		46 **coin**	/kɔɪn/	
7 **baby**	/beɪbi/		27 giving	/gɪvɪŋ/		47 soon	/suːn/	
8 board	/bɔːd/		28 **save**	/seɪv/		48 see	/siː/	
9 **beef**	/biːf/		29 thinking	/θɪŋkɪŋ/		49 **castle**	/kæsəl/	
10 **boot**	/buːt/		30 thought	/θɔːt/		50 easy	/iːzɪ/	
11 **bitter**	/bɪtə/		31 **teeth**	/tiːθ/		51 **cheese**	/tʃiːz/	
12 tube	/tjuːb/		32 this	/ðɪs/		52 **cage**	/keɪdʒ/	
13 job	/dʒɒb/		33 that	/ðæt/		53 **shoe**	/ʃuː/	
14 **mouth**	/maʊθ/		34 lower	/ləʊə/		54 **sugar**	/ʃʊgə/	
15 mother	/mʌðə/		35 with	/wɪð/		55 **washing**	/wɒʃɪŋ/	
16 **money**	/mʌnɪ/		36 talk	/tɔːk/		56 go	/gəʊ/	
17 **mouse**	/maʊs/		37 **wheel**	/wiːəl/		57 **church**	/tʃɜːtʃ/	
18 measure	/meʒə/		38 night	/naɪt/		58 **catching**	/kætʃɪŋ/	
19 summer	/sʌmə/		39 **sheet**	/ʃiːt/		59 **watch**	/wɒtʃ/	
20 wisdom	/wɪzdəm/		40 **door**	/dɔː/		60 July	/dʒəlaɪ/	
						61 **edge**	/edʒ/	

Clusters

Word		Score	Word		Score	Word		Score
62 play	/pleɪ/		69 smile	/smaɪəl/		76 stop	/stɒp/	
63 smoke	/sməʊk/		70 trip	/trɪp/		77 cloud	/klaʊd/	
64 three	/θriː/		71 shrugged	/ʃrəgd/		78 grass	/græs/	
65 snow	/snəʊ/		72 screen	/skriːn/		79 brown	/braʊn/	
66 sky	/skaɪ/		73 slope	/sləʊp/		80 free	/friː/	
67 sweet	/swiːt/		74 blue	/bluː/		81 draw	/drɔː/	
68 present	/prezənt/		75 flower	/flaʊə/		82 crown	/kraʊn/	
						83 glasses	/glæsɪz/	

Multisyllabic words

Word		Score	Word		Score
84 supporting	/sə'pɔːtɪŋ/		91 understanding	/ʌndə'stændɪŋ/	
85 customer	/'kʌstəmə/		92 electricity	/elek'trɪsɪtɪ/	
86 musicians	/mjuː'zɪʃənz/		93 sophisticated	/sə'fɪstəkeɪtɪd/	
87 gardener	/'gɑːdənə/		94 investigation	/ɪnvestɪ'geɪʃən/	
88 television	/telɪ'vɪʒən/		95 anniversary	/ænɪ'vɜːsərɪ/	
89 dictionary	/'dɪkʃənərɪ/		96 responsibility	/rəspɒnsɪ'bɪlɪtɪ/	
90 helicopter	/helɪ'kɒptə/				

ANALYSIS CHARTS

Add up the scores for each sound in each word position and note the total on the analysis chart.

WI	word initial position
WM	word medial position
WF	word final position
Cl	in a consonant cluster
Multi	in a multisyllabic word

Consonants

	p	b	m	t	d	n	f	v	θ	ð	s	z	ʃ	ʒ	tʃ	dʒ	k	g	j	w	l	r	h
WI																							
WM																							
WF																							
Cl																							
Multi																							

Vowels

Short	ɪ	e	æ	ɒ	ʊ	ʌ	ə
Long	iː	ɑː	uː	ɔː	ɜː		
Diphthongs	eɪ	aɪ	aʊ	əʊ	ɪə	eə	ʊə

Notes

Routledge Taylor & Francis Group   P This page may be photocopied for instructional use only. *Lemon & Lime Library* © R Palmer & A Protopapas 2008

1

pen

2

hoping

cap

tip

5

paper

6

bag

baby

board

beef

boot

11

bitter

12

tube

job

mouth

mother

---

money

mouse

---

measure

19

summer

20

wisdom

feet

fish

23

fourth

24

laughing

lorry

---

van

giving

save

thinking

---

thought

teeth

---

this

that

lower

with

---

talk

wheel

---

night

sheet

door

red

---

nose

looking

younger

45

zone

46

coin

soon

---

see

castle

easy

cheese

cage

shoe

sugar

55

washing

56

go

church

---

catching

watch

July

edge

---

play

smoke

---

three

snow

---

sky

sweet

---

present

smile

trip

71

shrugged

72

screen

slope

---

blue

flower

---

stop

cloud

grass

brown

free

draw

---

crown

83

glasses

84

supporting

customer

musicians

gardener

television

dictionary

---

helicopter

91

understanding

92

electricity

93

sophisticated

94

investigation

anniversary

responsibility

1

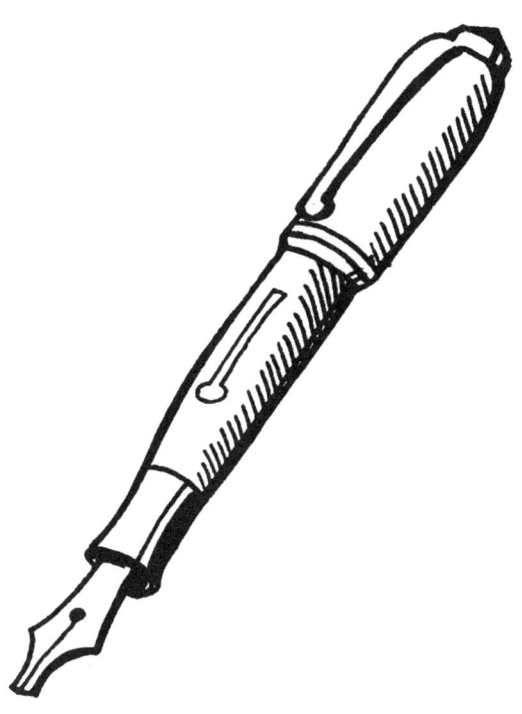

3

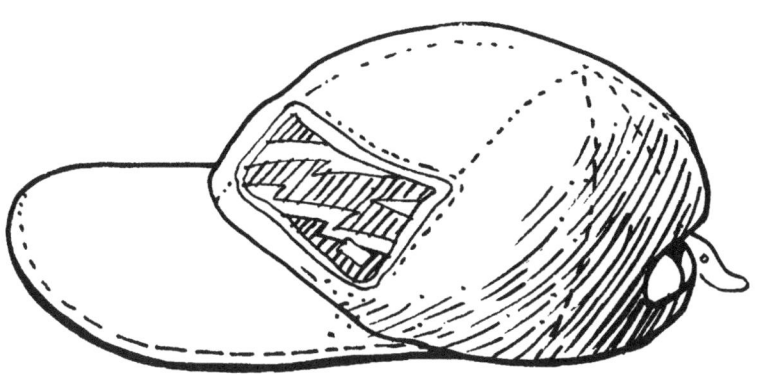

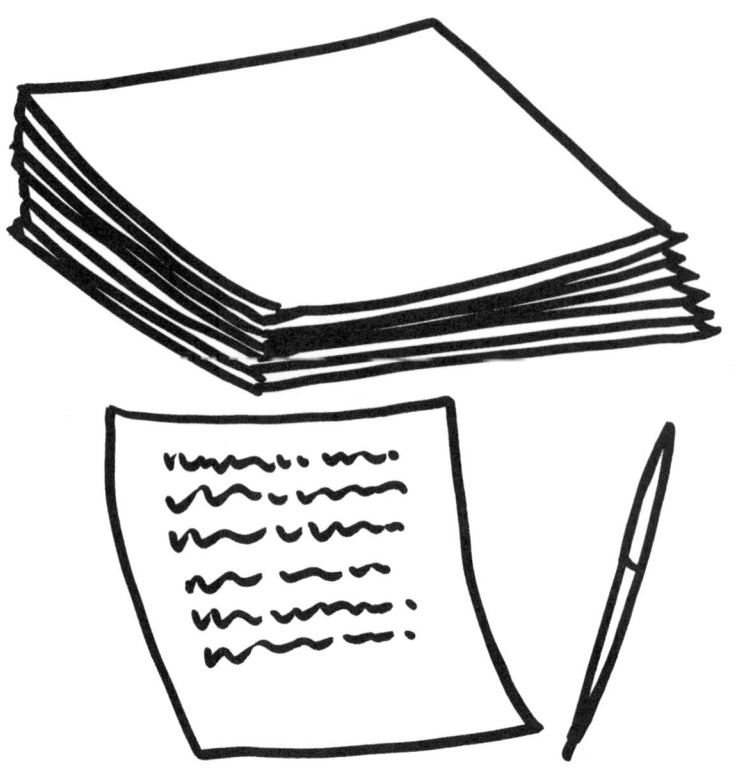

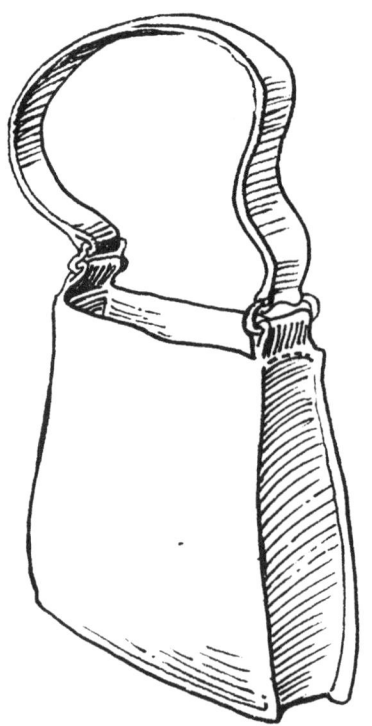

7

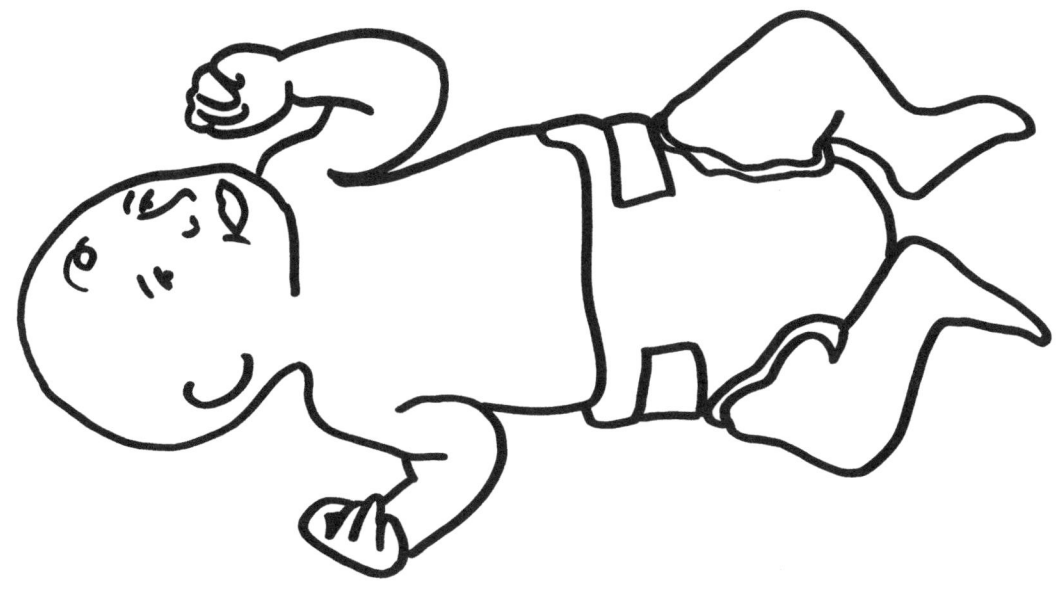

9

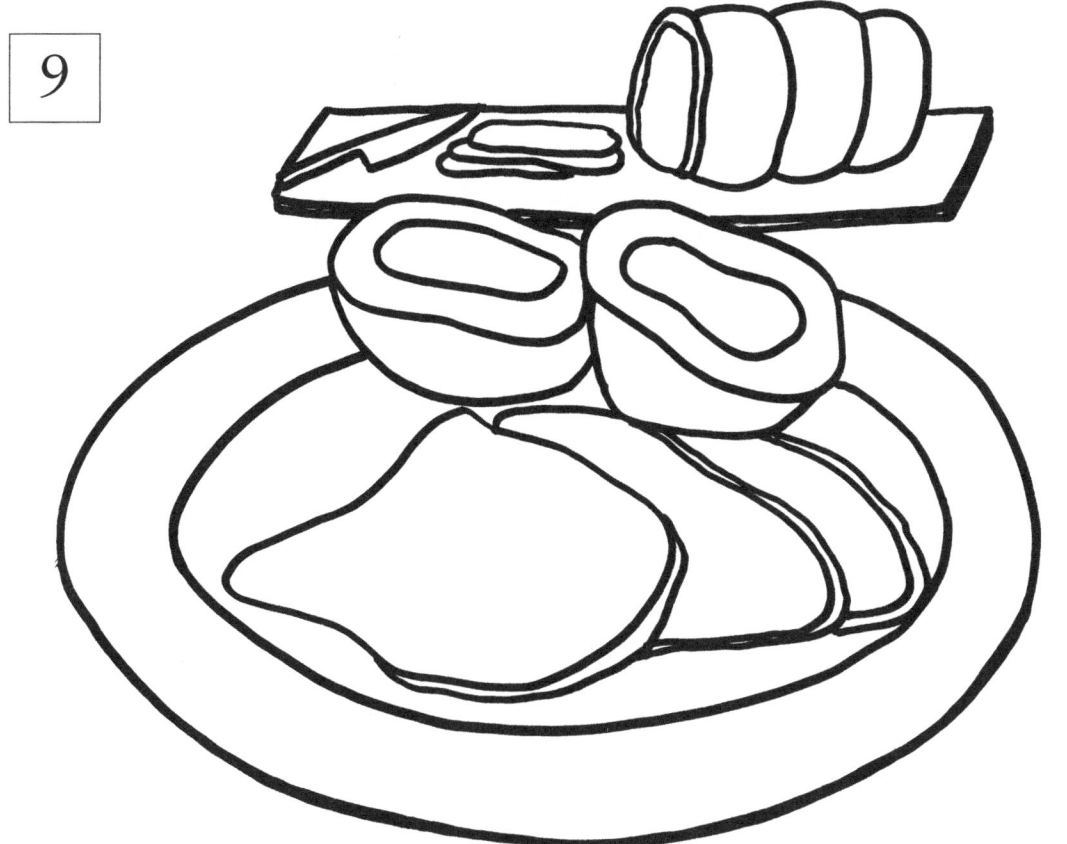

10

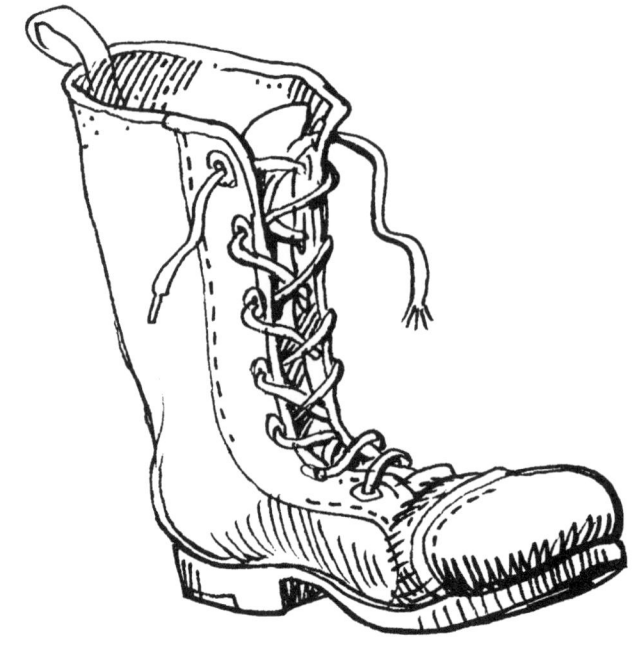

11

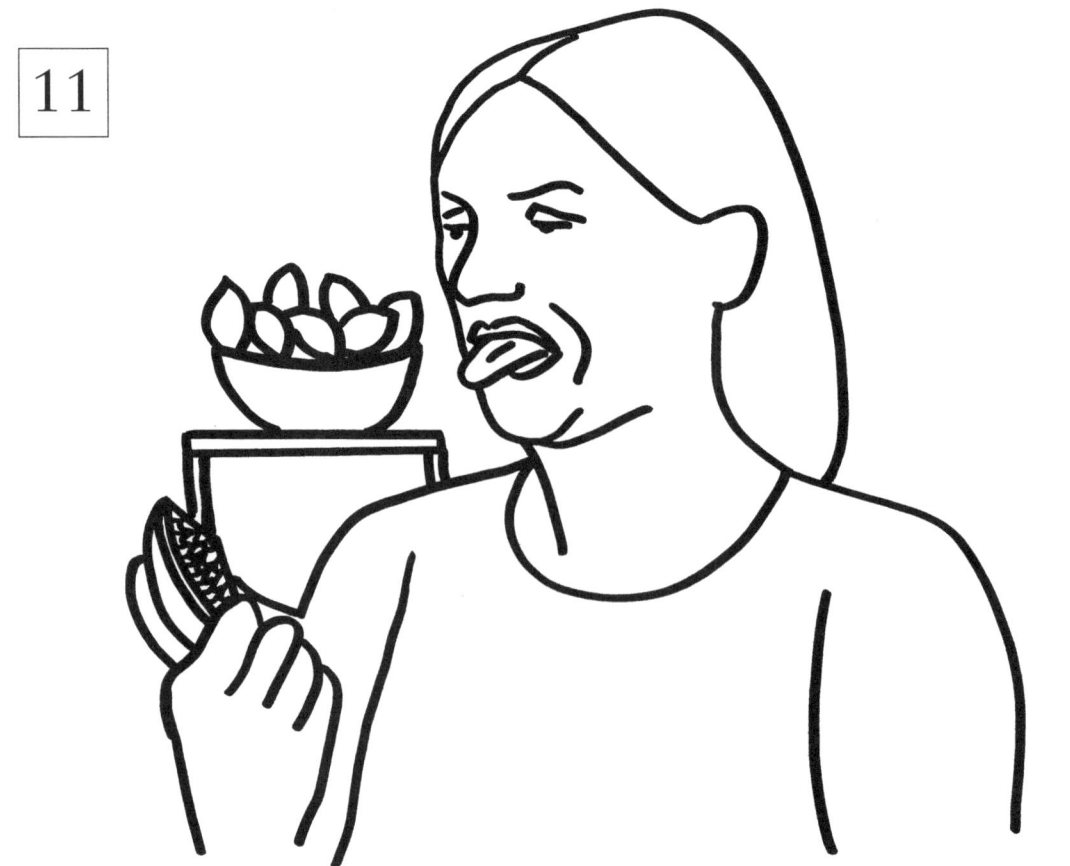

14

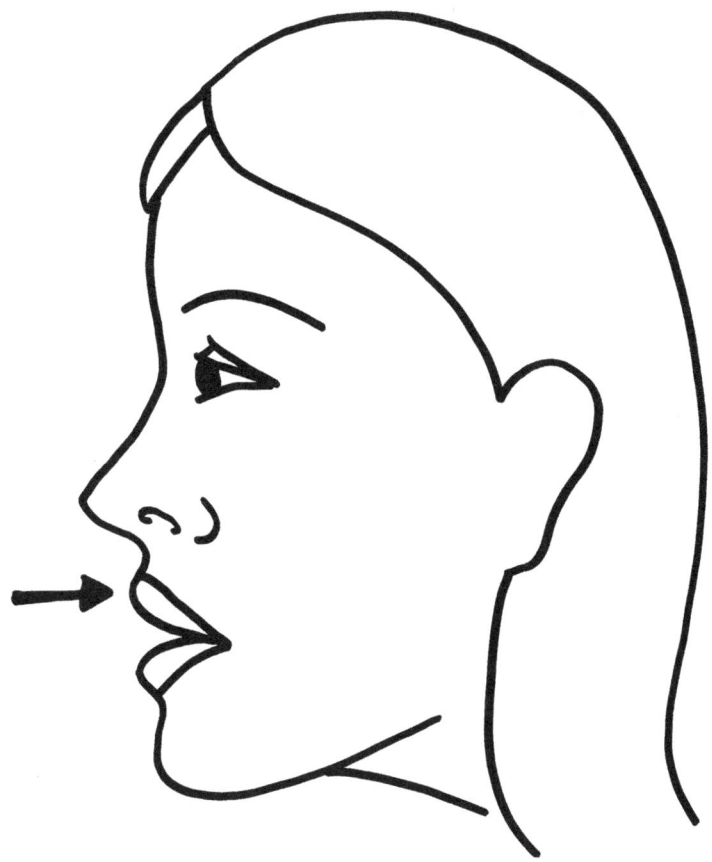

16

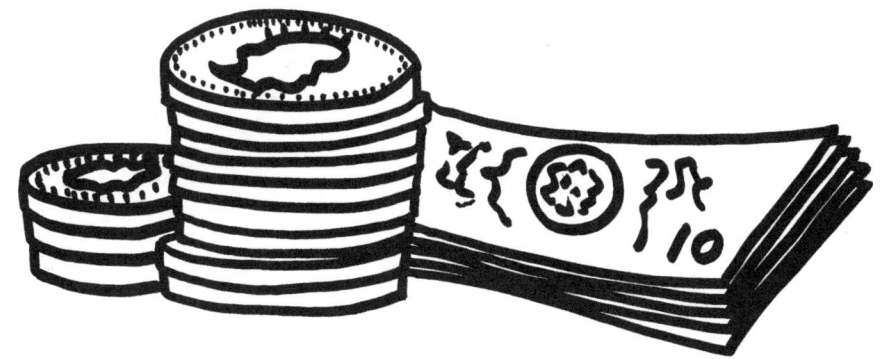

17

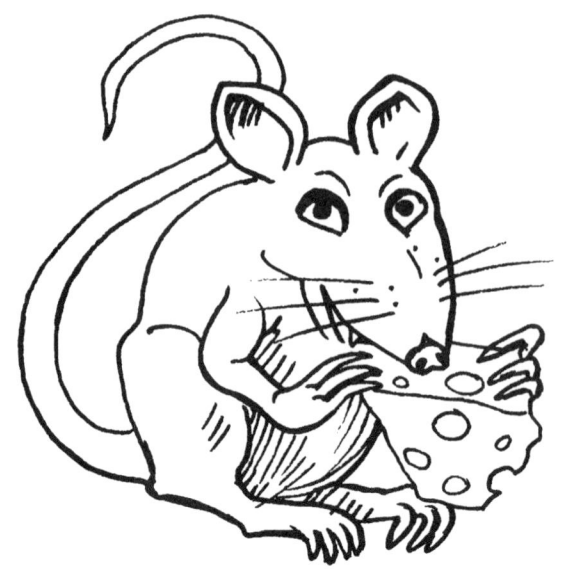

21

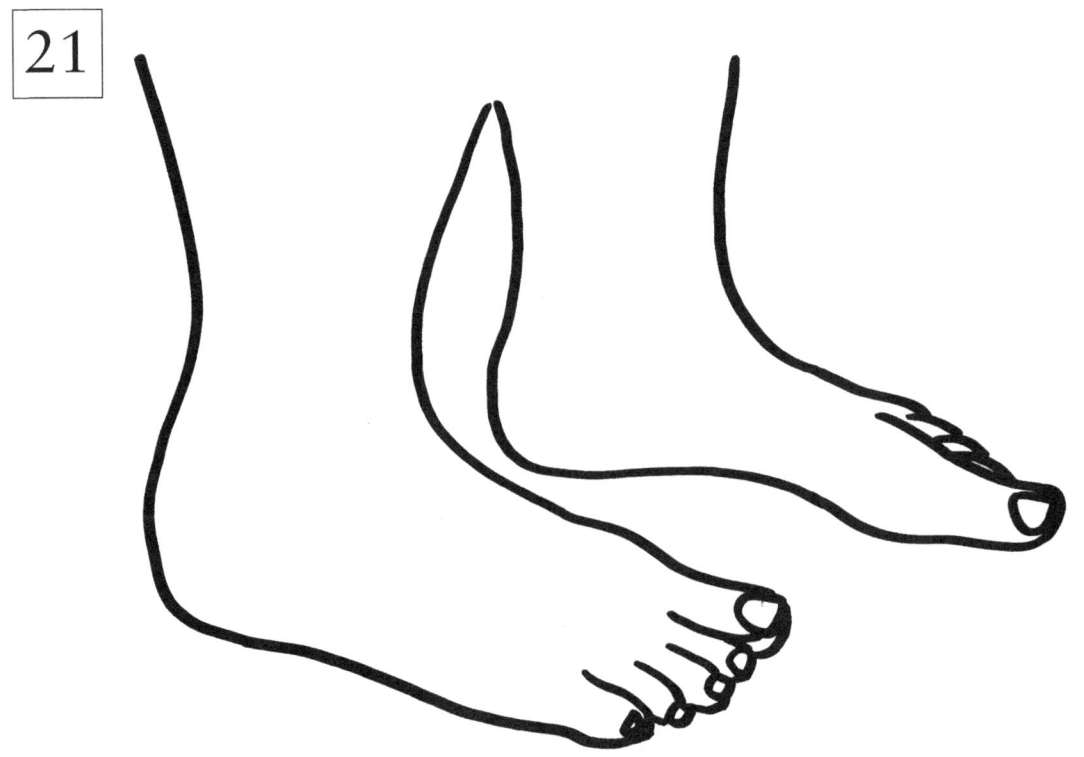

22

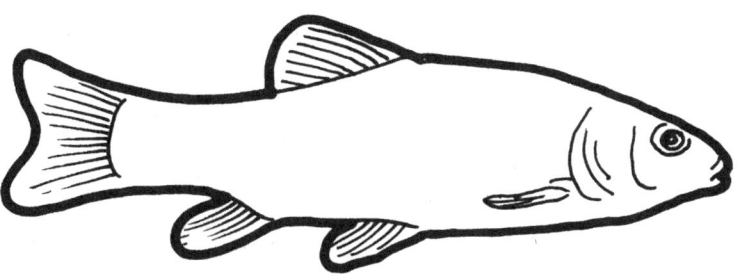

23

4th

24

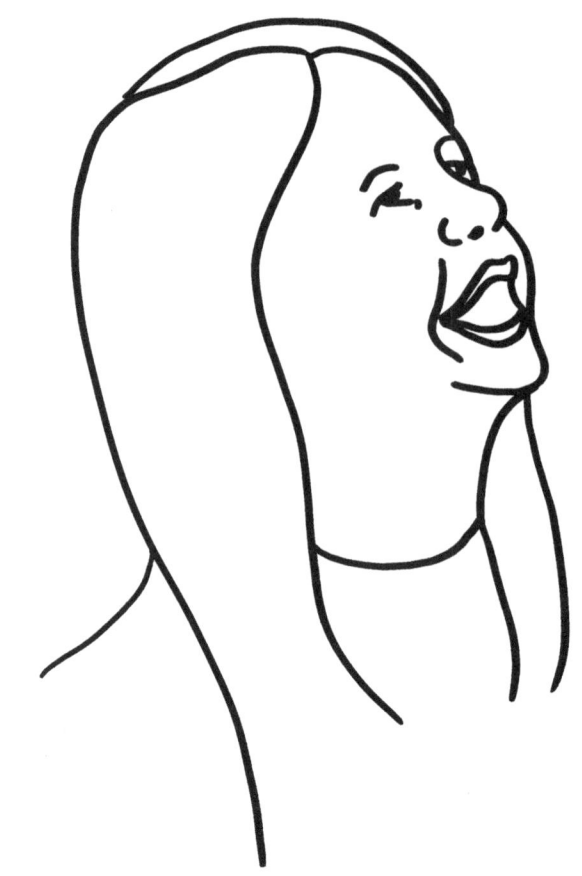

25

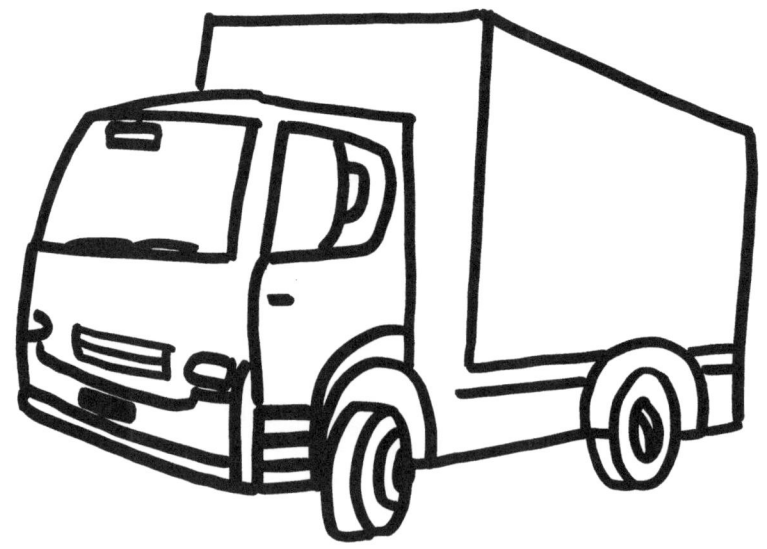

26

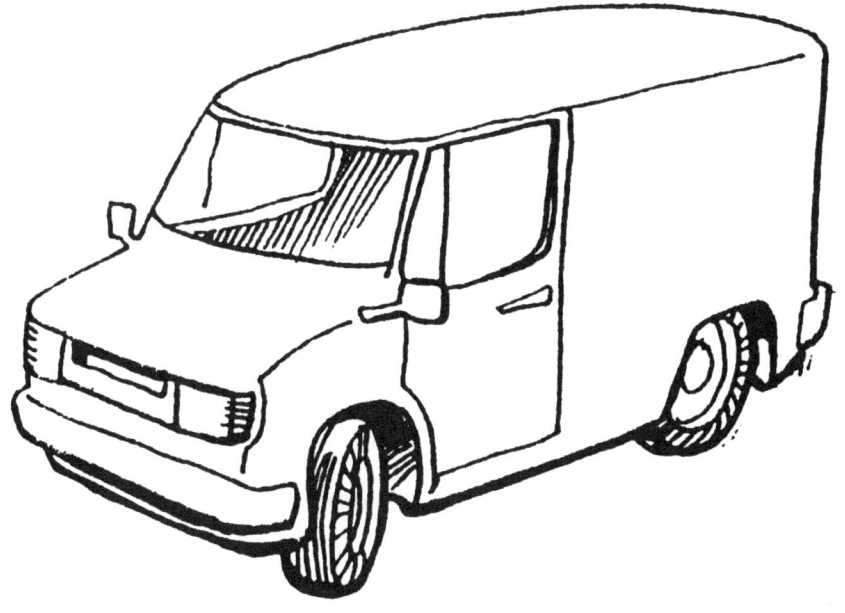

28

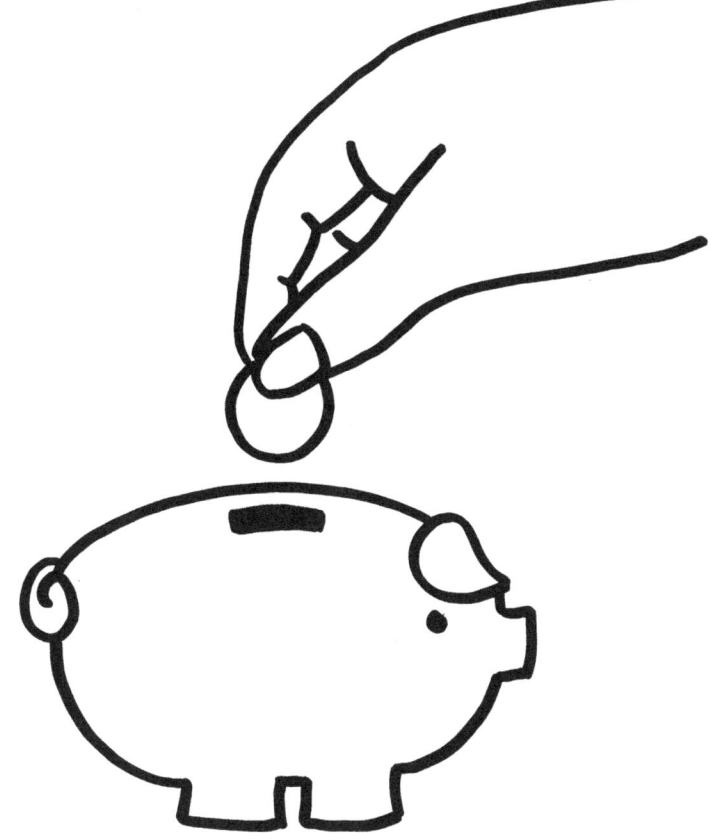

31

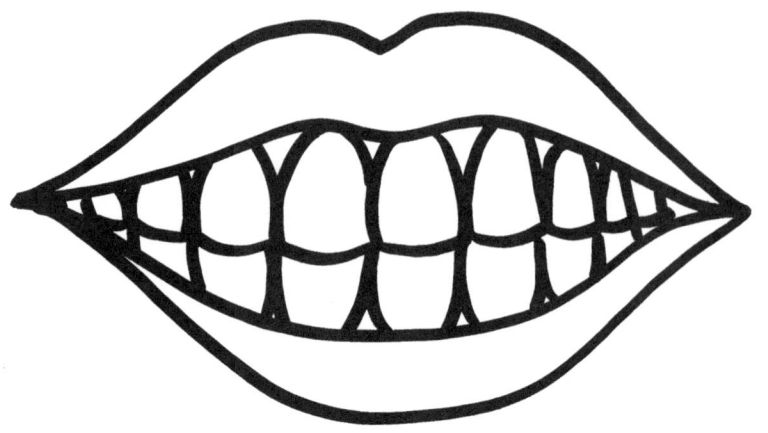

37

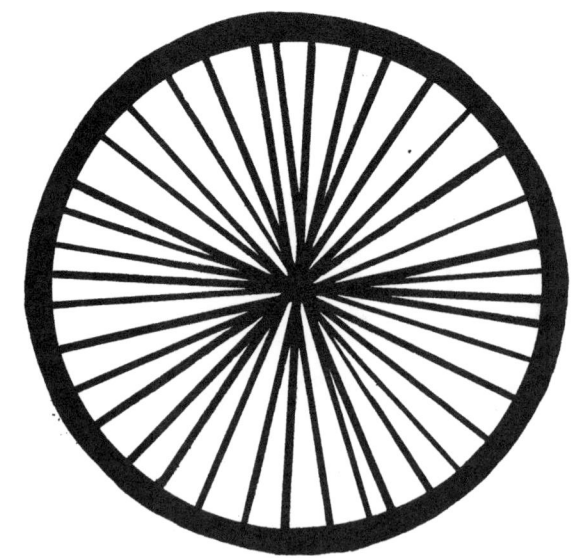

39

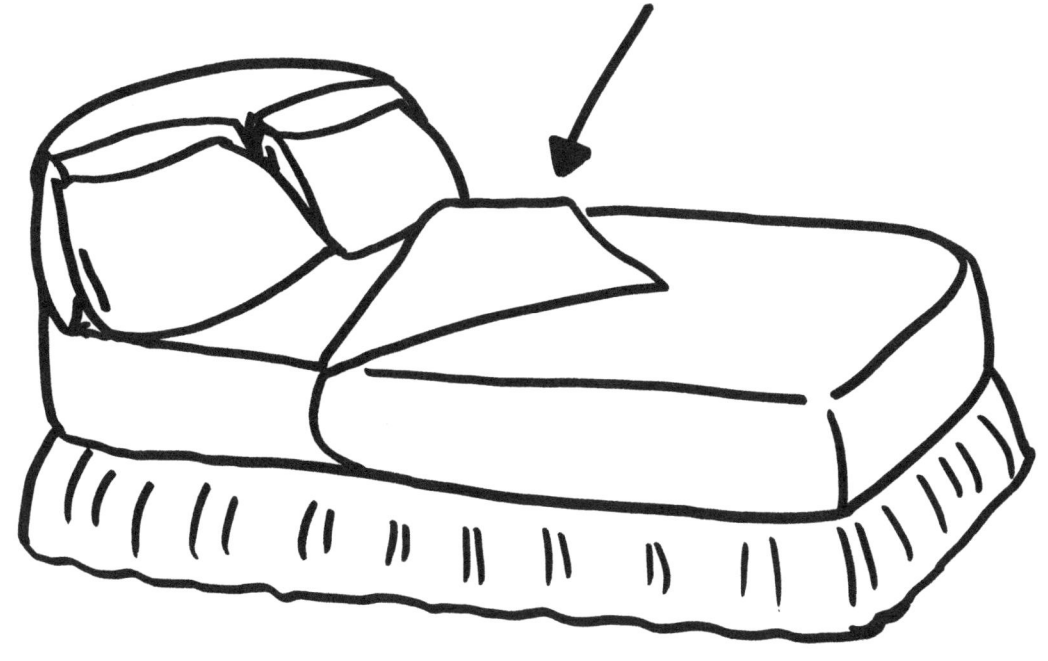

40

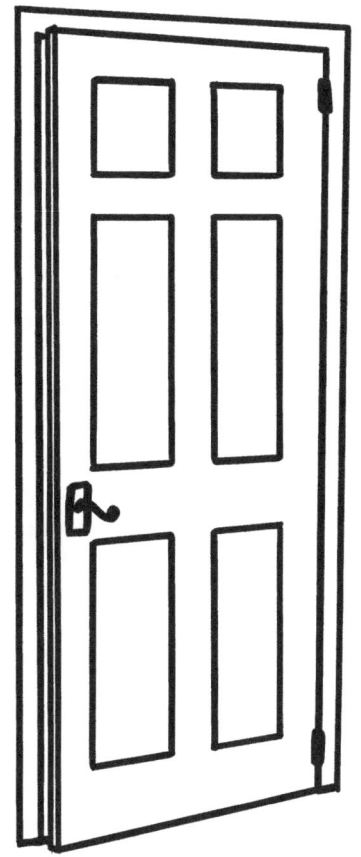

42

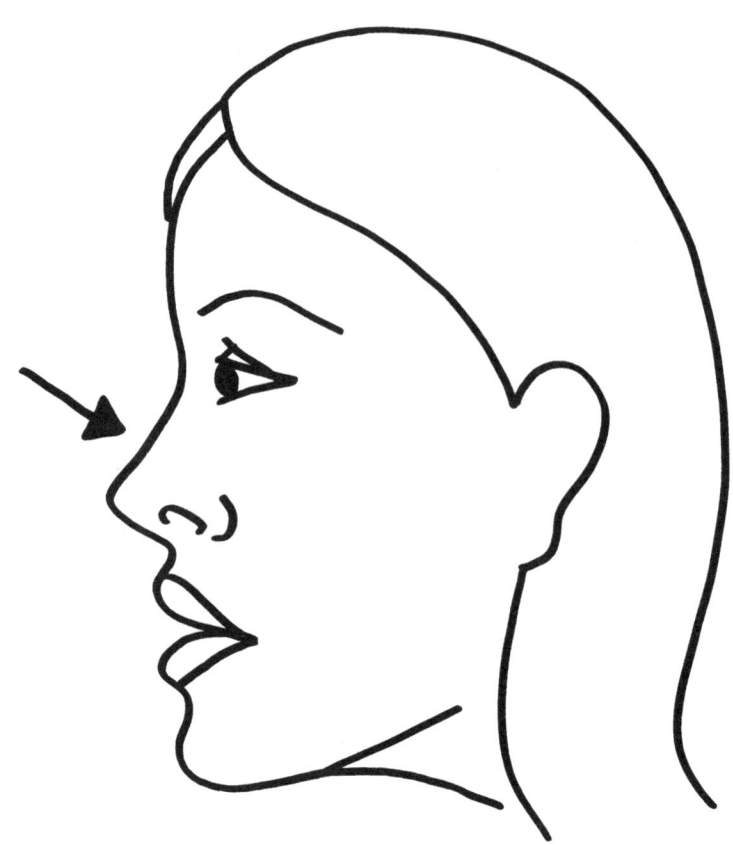

46

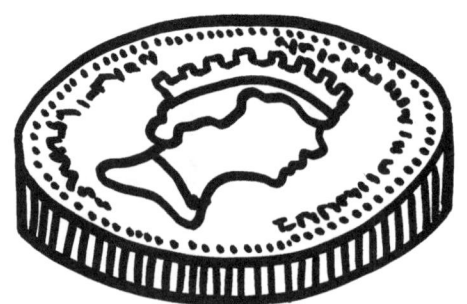

49

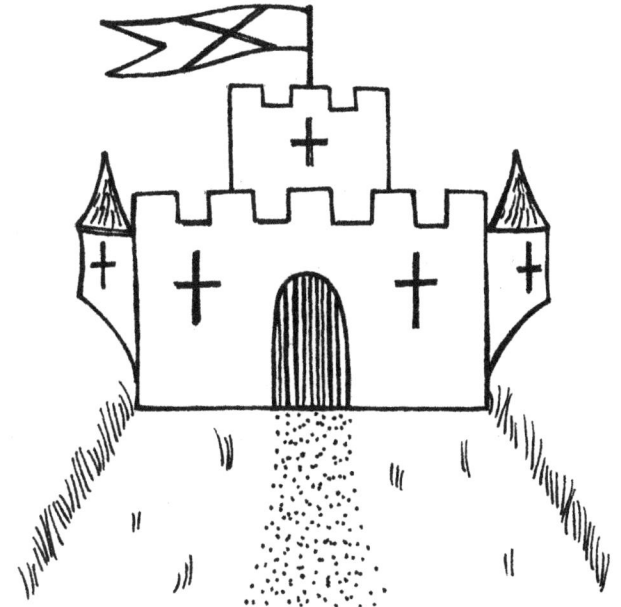

51

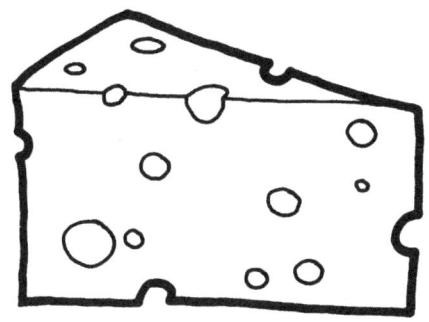

52

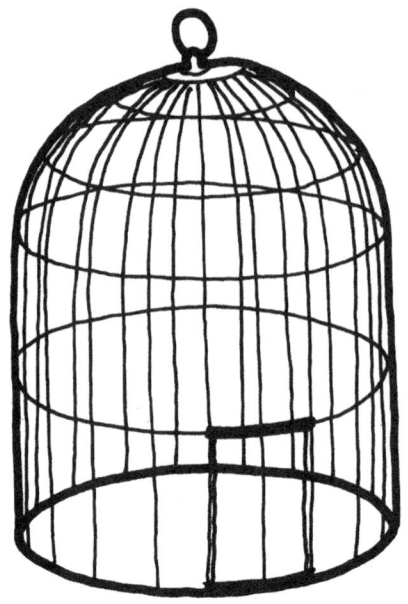

53

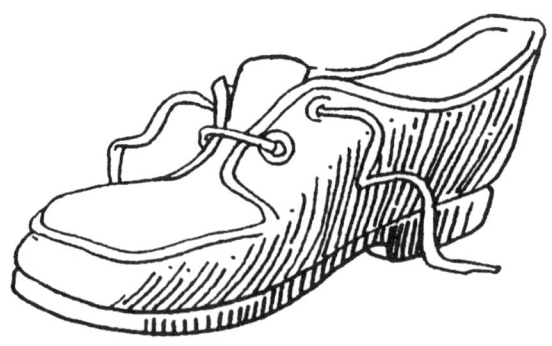

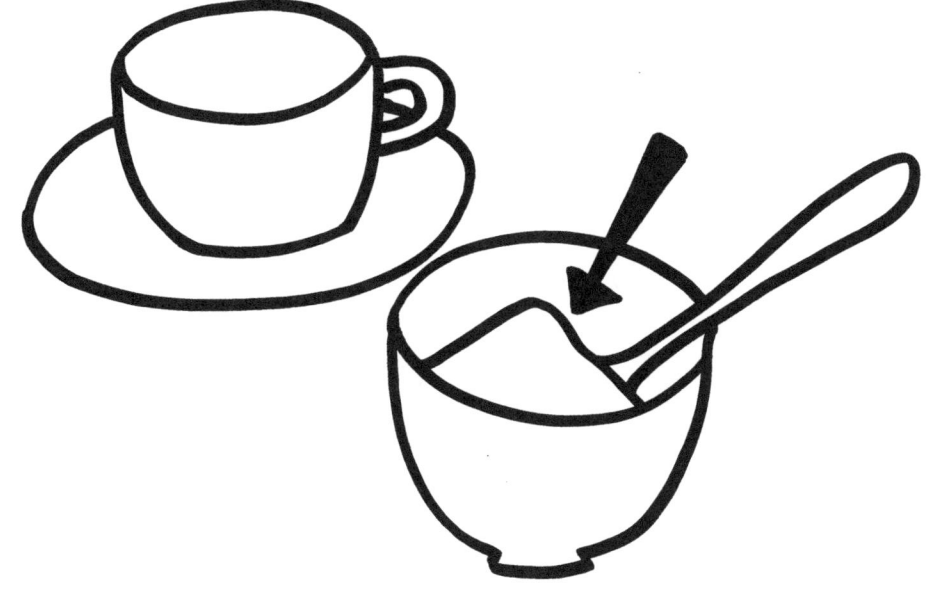

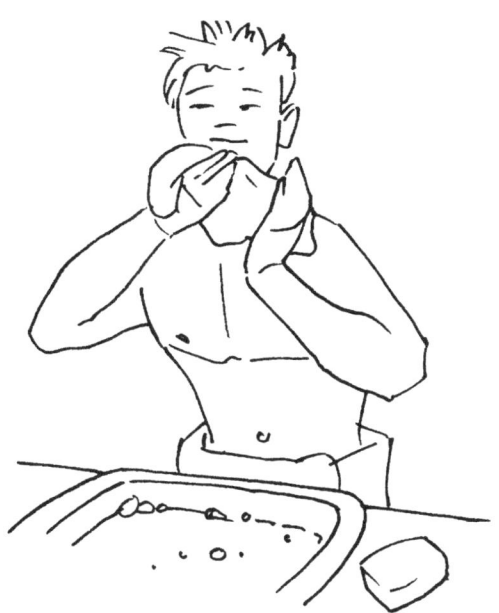

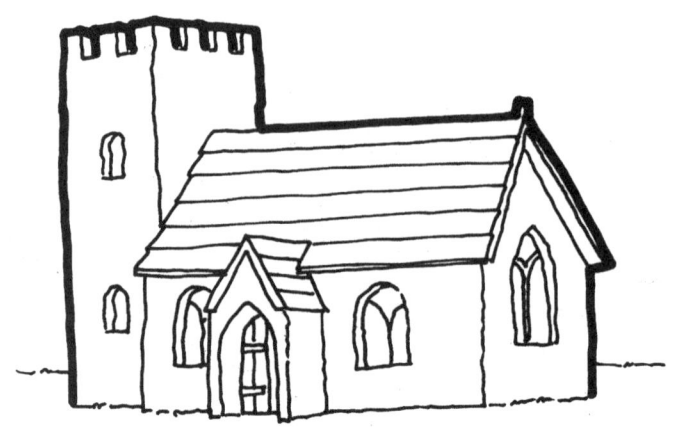

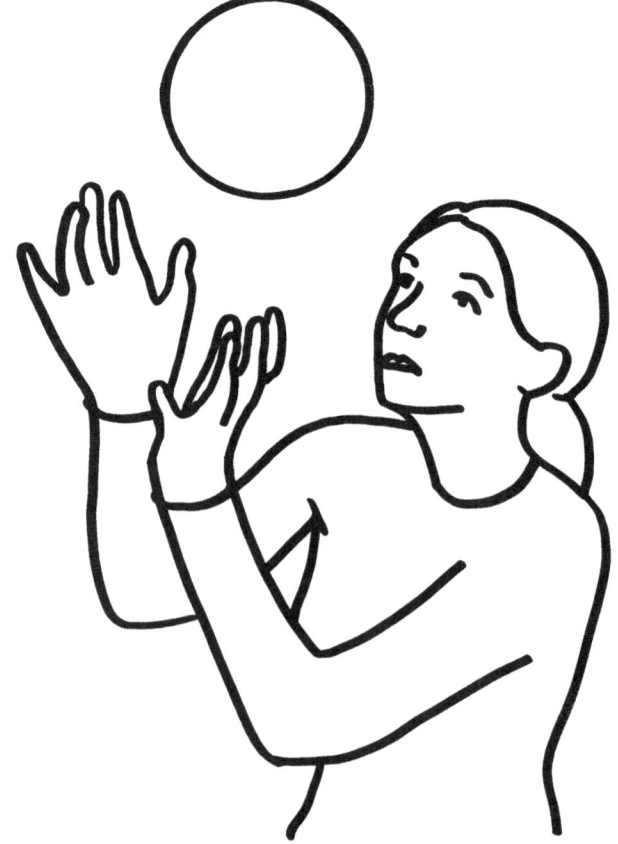

59

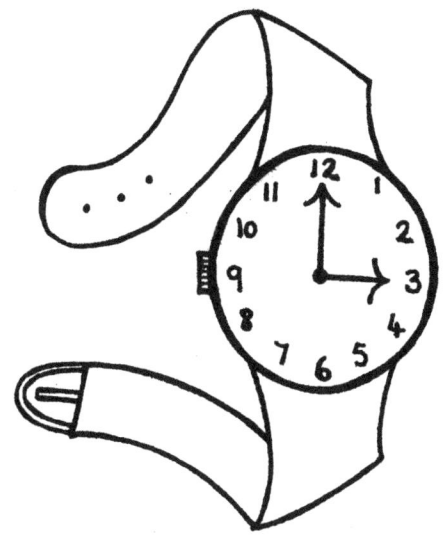

61

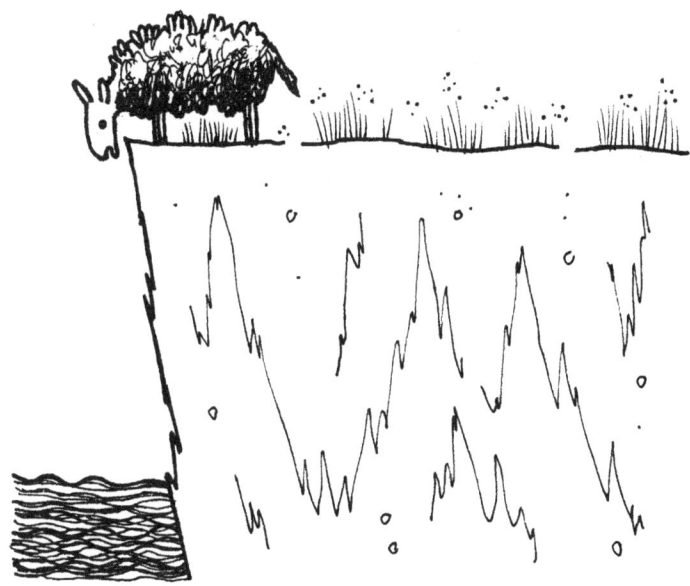

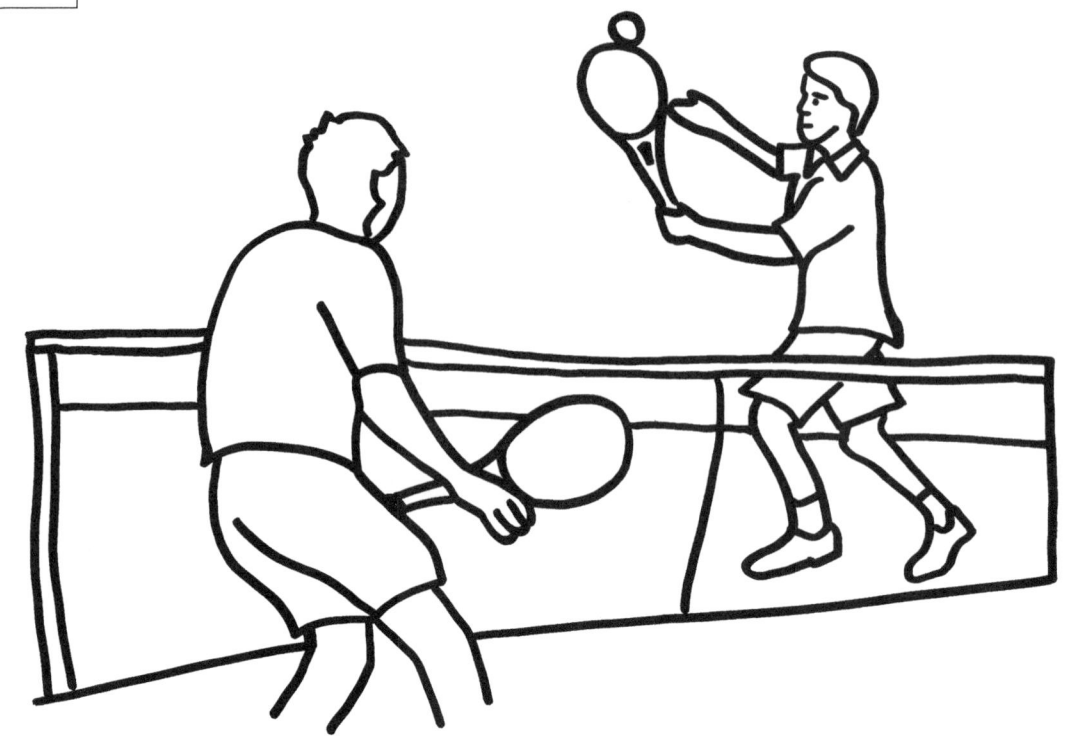

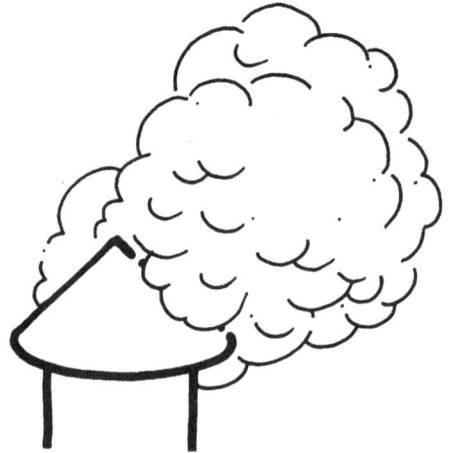

64

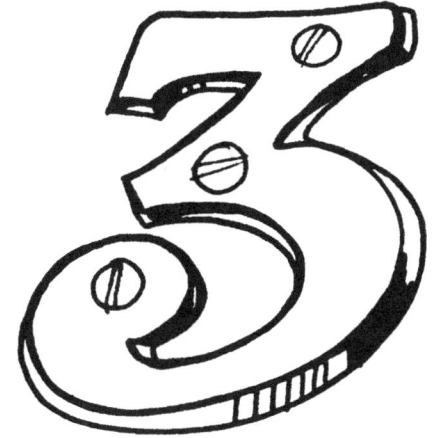

65

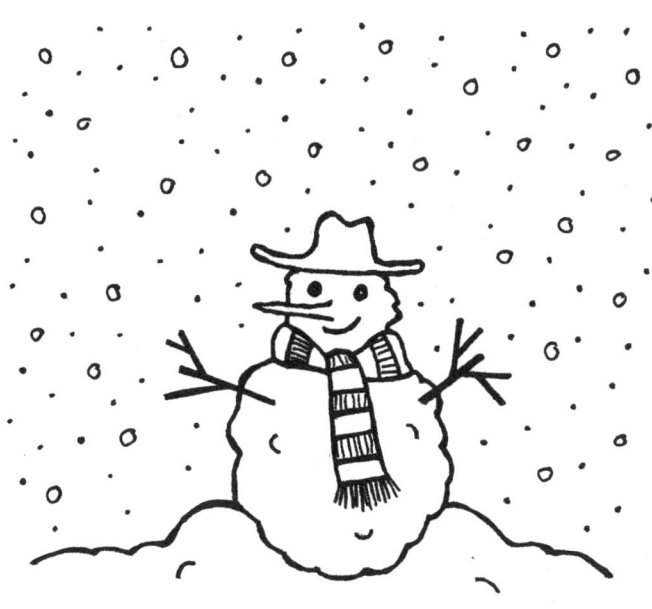

66

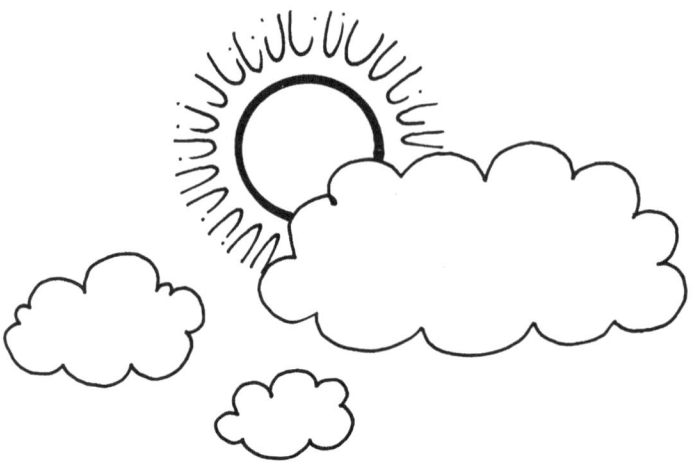

67

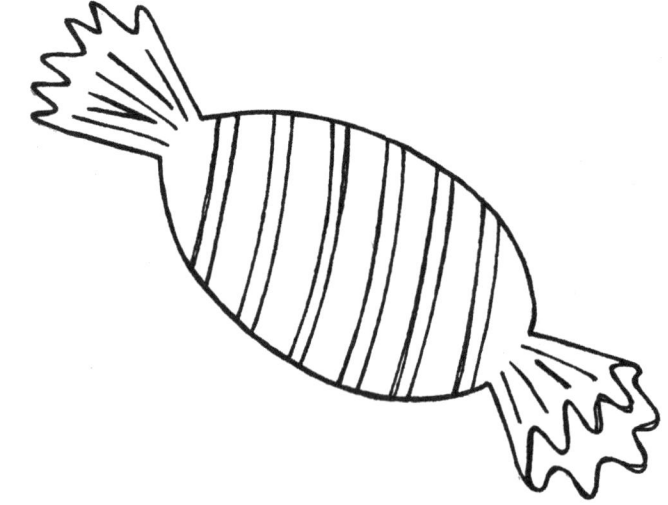

69

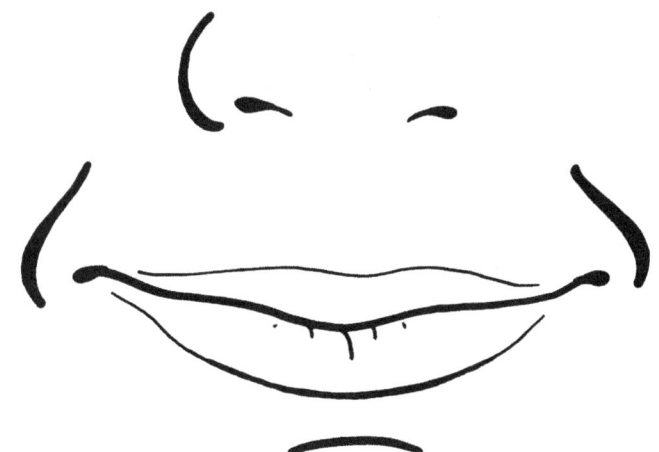

72

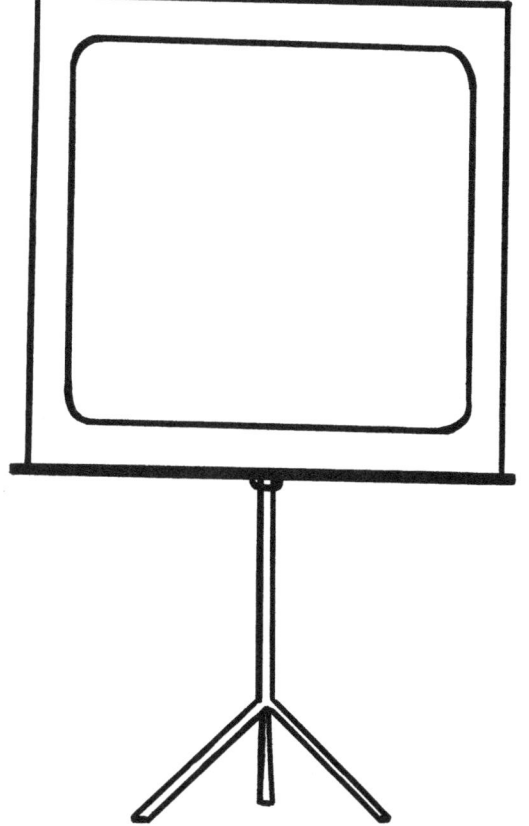

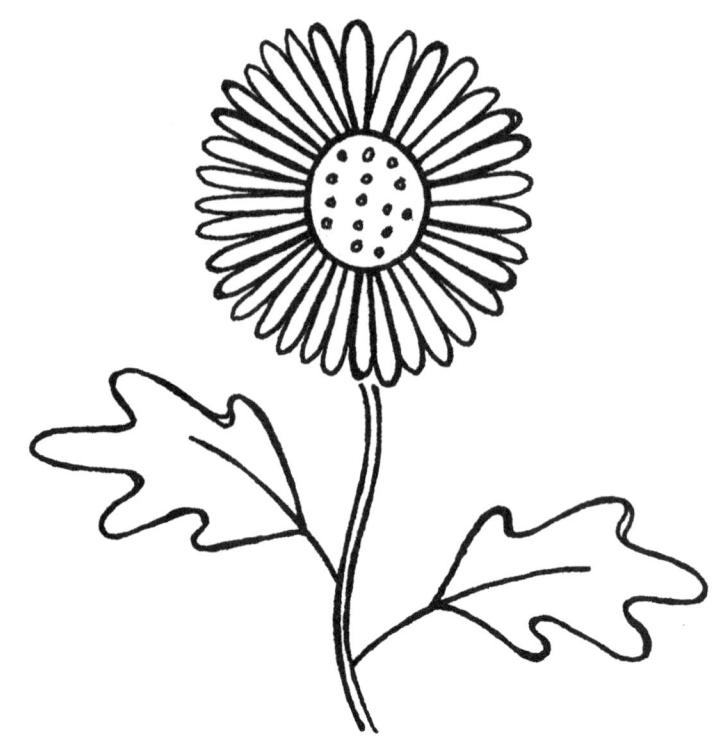

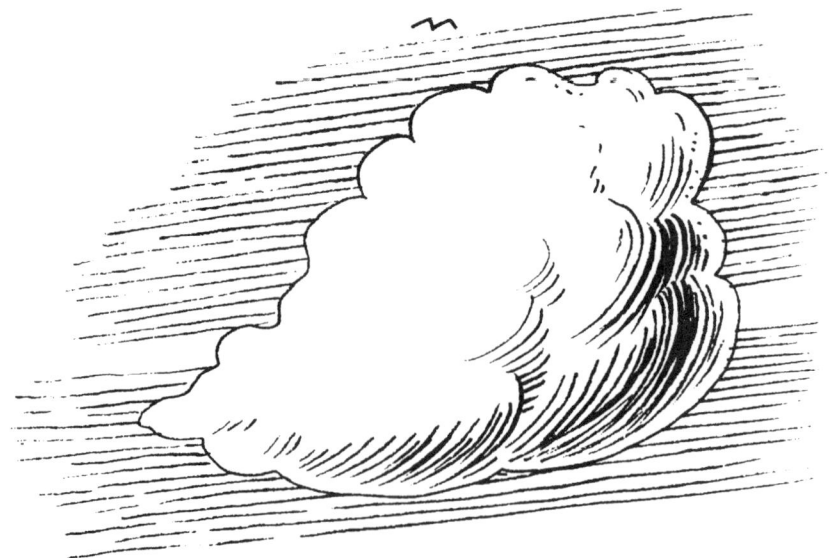

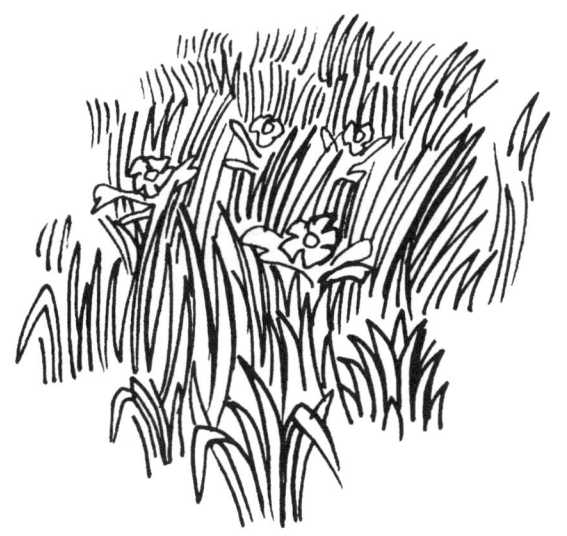

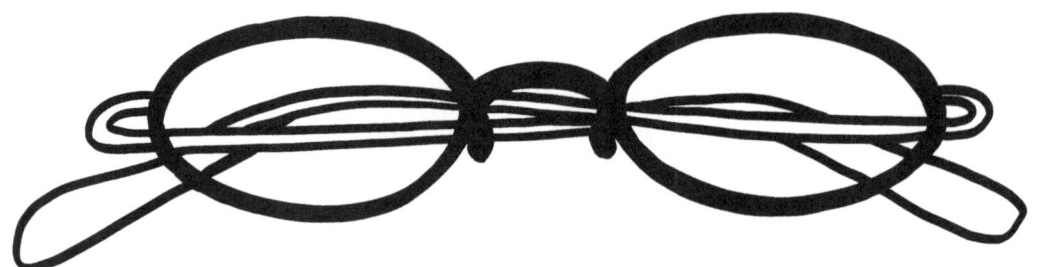

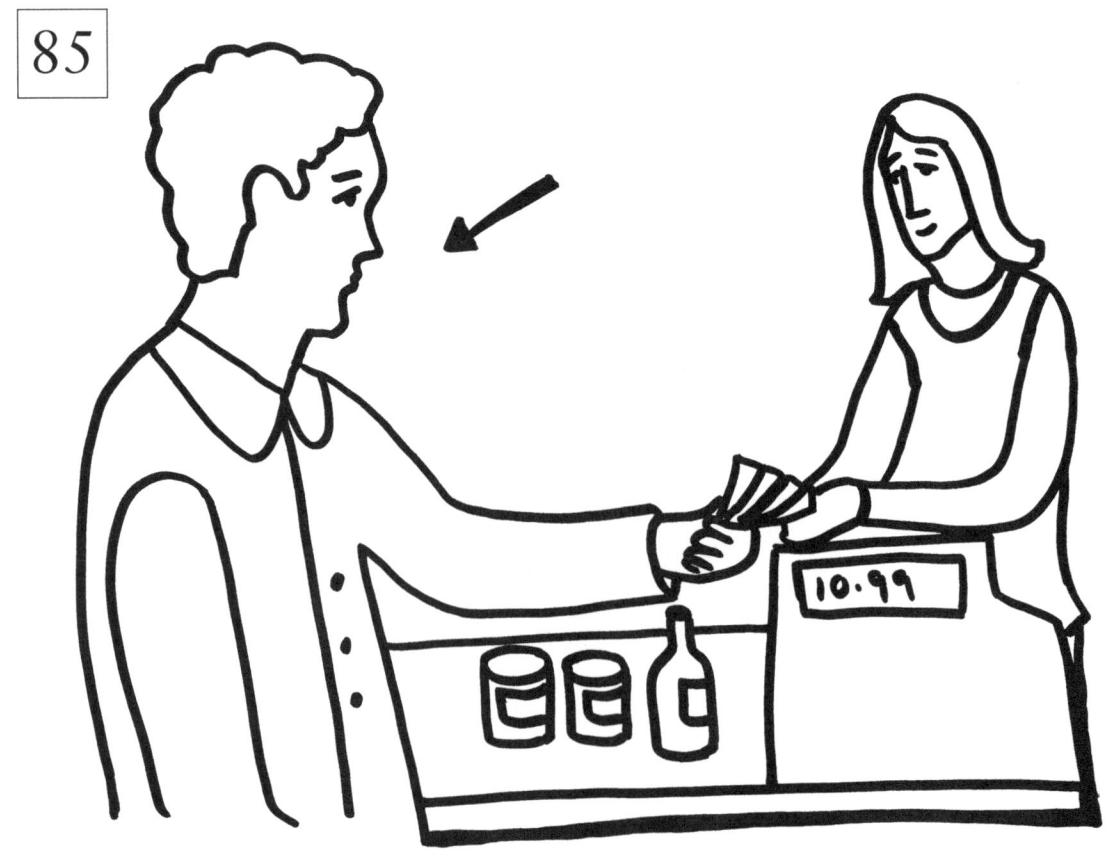

86

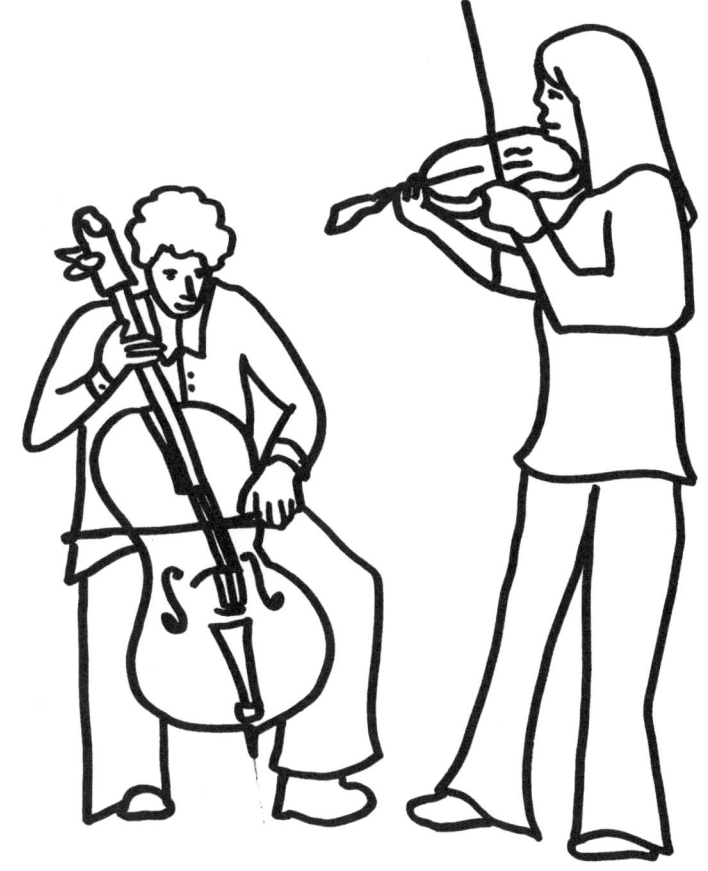

88

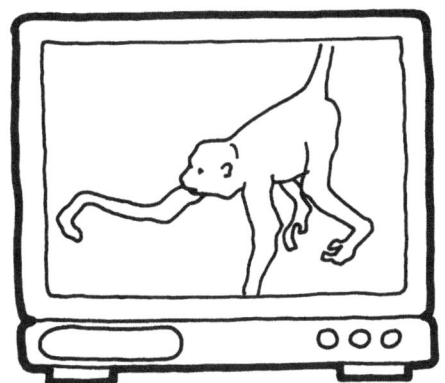

PART III
Resource pack

LEMON & LIME LIBRARY OF SOUNDS & WORDS

How the Lemon & Lime Library of words is organised

The sounds and words in this chapter are available for use from the following photocopiable pages (pp102–250). They are organised by level:

LEVEL 1

Single sounds in isolation.

LEVEL 2

Level 2 CV and VC words are presented with words targeting different phonemes in different lists. Target phonemes made in the same place are presented on one page. For example, lists of words with bilabial targets can all be found on the same page. If there are more than three sounds that are made at a single place, lists are further subdivided according to the manner of articulation: for example, alveolar stops and alveolar fricatives. Lists of voiceless targets appear before voiced targets, and CV words are presented above VC words with the same target sound.

LEVEL 3

For level 3, all phonemes are printed with the vowel /æ/ in CVCV to be practised up to ten times each (Lange *et al*, 2000).

LEVEL 4

Level 4 presents alternating consonants in CVCV strings. The Lemon & Lime Library offers a range of alternations between place, manner and voicing.

LEVEL 5

For Level 5, short words are presented with one target phoneme per page organised from front to back sounds. Voiceless targets are also presented before voiced ones. The lists are further subdivided into the word position of the target sound, in order of word initial, word medial and word final positions. Words with the target appearing in a consonant cluster appear at the end of level 5.

LEVEL 6

In Level 6, multisyllabic words are presented with a single sound target per page as for Level 5 words. All targets appear only in word initial position. For Level 6, the lists are subdivided into the number of syllables in the word in order of the number of syllables, that is, lists of 2 syllable words precede lists of 3 syllable words and so on up to 5 or 6 syllables.

Notes on the illustrations

1   The illustrated words are presented in bold in the tables.

2   Illustrations that appear together on a page all come from the same word table. Thicker lines are used to frame words within the same target sound in a different word position.

3   Pictures representing different sounds are presented in separate boxes.

LEVEL 1 Single sounds in isolation

LEVEL 1 lists all the sounds of the English language in isolation. Each sound is presented orthographically and phonetically.

Consonants

Orthography	p	b	m	f	v	th (three)	th (the)	t	d	n	s	z
Phonetics	p	b	m	f	v	θ	ð	t	d	n	s	z
Orthography	sh	measure	ch	j	k		g		ng	w	r	l	y	h
Phonetics	ʃ	ʒ	tʃ	dʒ	k		g		ŋ	w	r	l	j	h

Vowels

Short	ɪ	e	æ	ɒ	ʌ	ʊ	ə	
	pin	pen	pan	on	bun	hood	pepper	
Long	iː	uː	ɜː	ɑː	ɔː			
	see	Sue	sir	car	poor			
Diphthongs	eɪ	aɪ	ɔɪ	əʊ	aʊ	ɪə	eə	ʊə
	gate	eye	boy	toe	how	ear	hair	manure

LEVEL 2 CV and VC words

LEVEL 2 lists words made up of all consonants in the English language either before or after a vowel sound. These lists can be photocopied for speech practice. Imageable words are also presented in picture form.

CV and VC words sorted according to vowel

p	b	m
pea	**bee**	me
pa	baa	ma
poor	boo	**moo**
pie	bore	more
pay	bay	may
pear	**bear**	mare
	bye	my
up	**bow**	mow
ape	boy	
	beer	

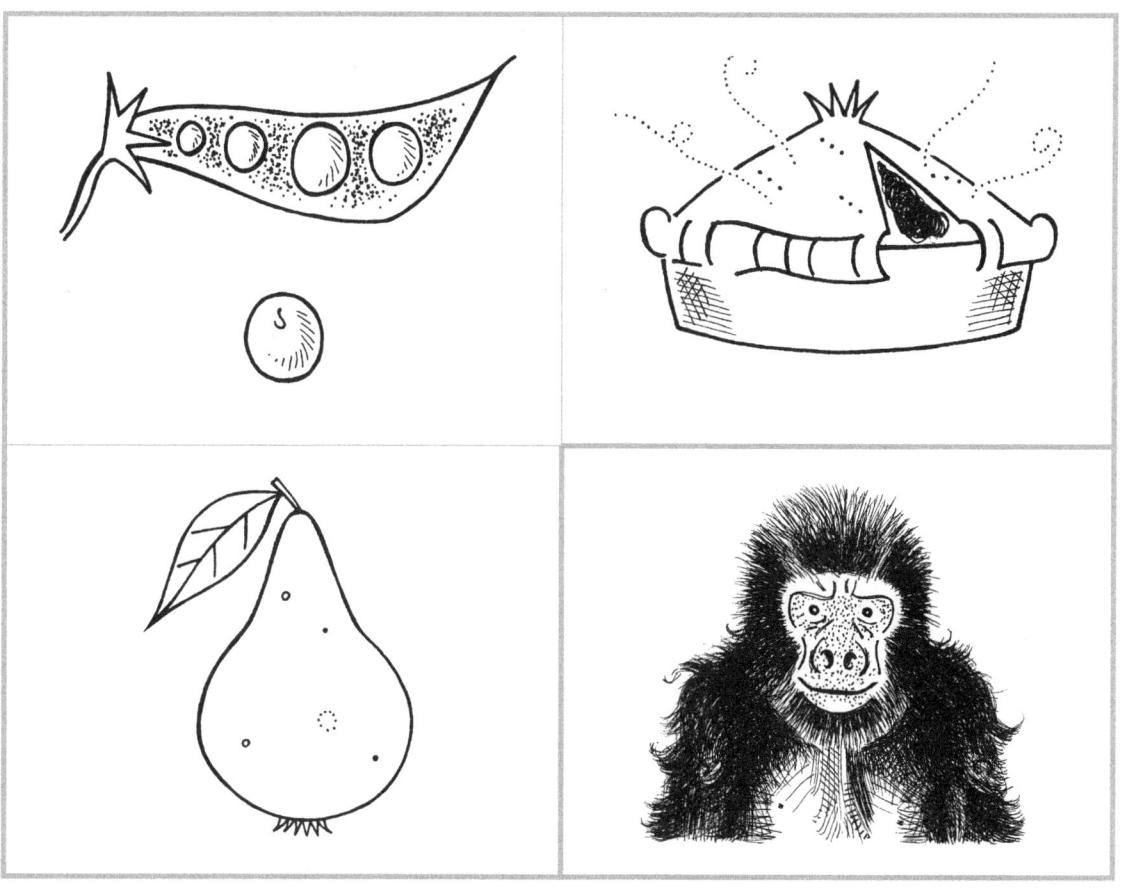

pea, pie, pear   ape

CV WI /b/ and /m/

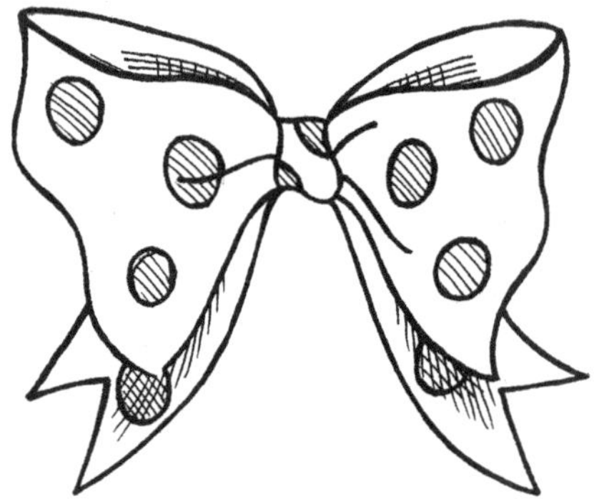

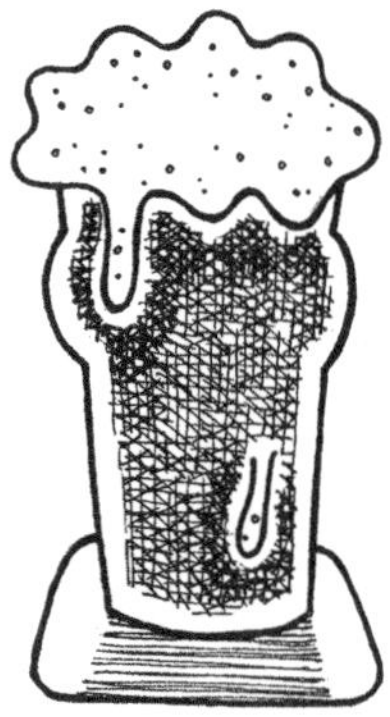

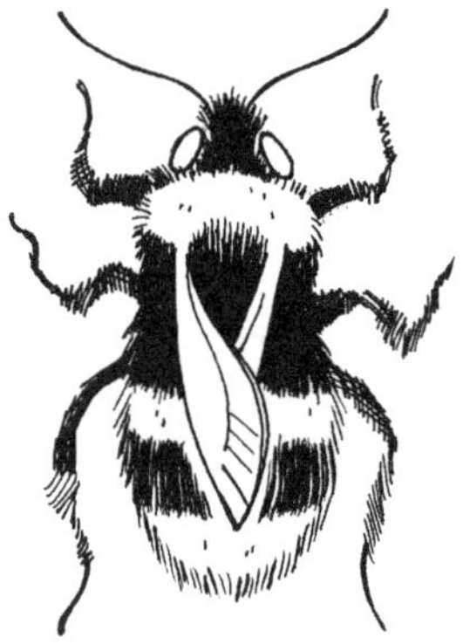

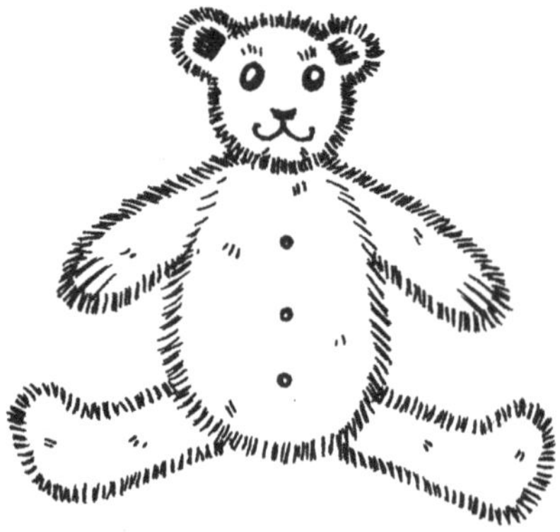

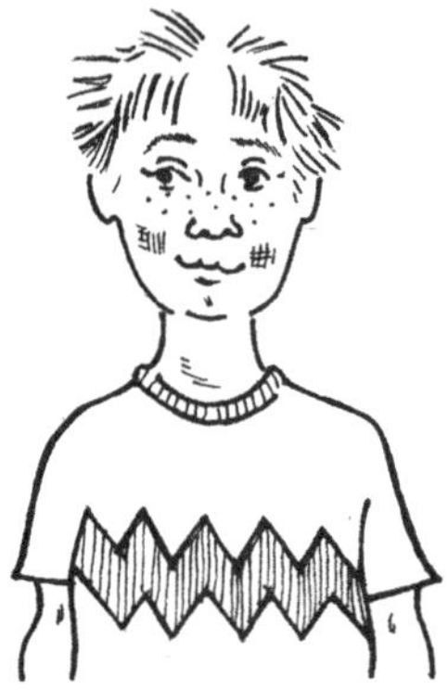

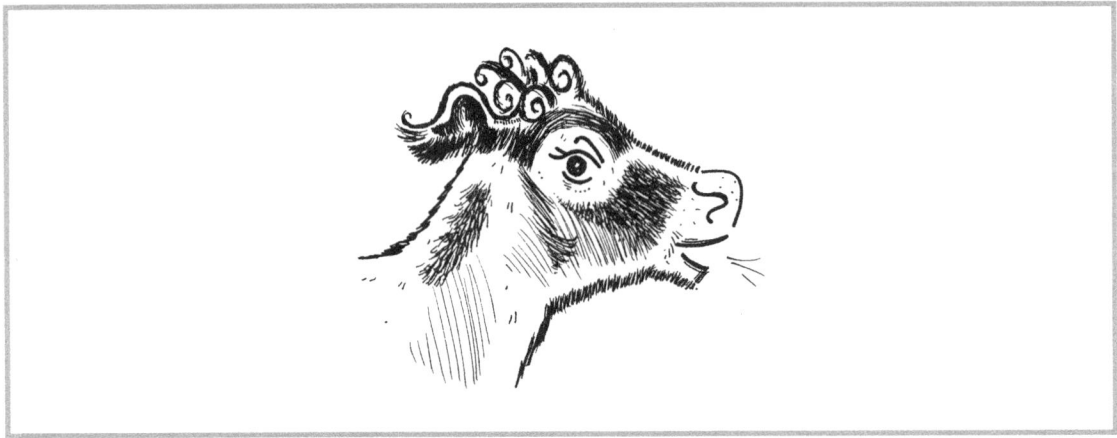

bee, bear, bow, boy, beer   moo

Labiodental and interdental sounds
(with teeth)

f	th as in think	th as in this
fee	**thigh**	the
far	thaw	they
four		
fur		
foe		
fay		
fair		

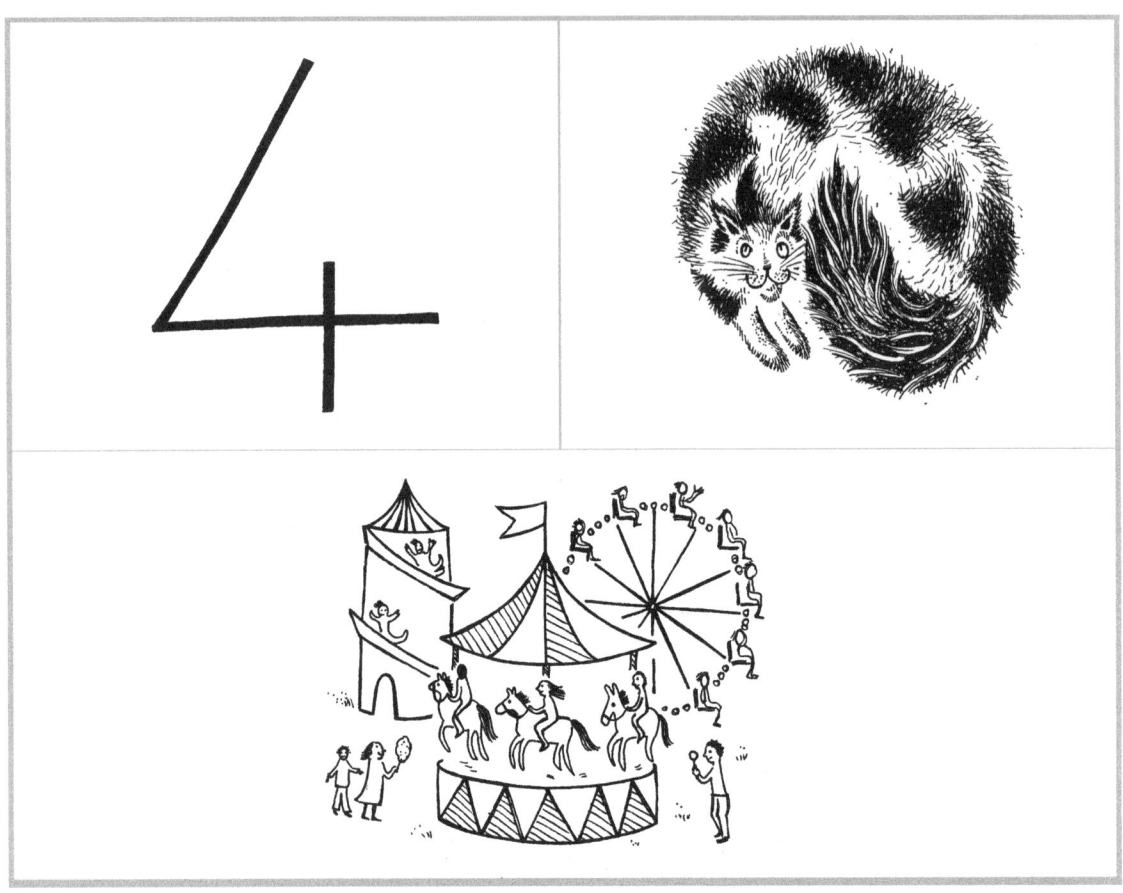

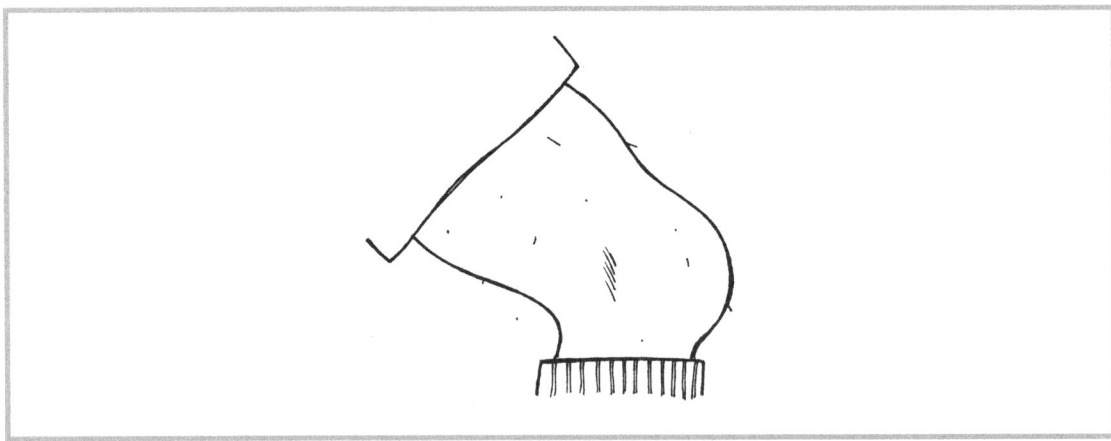

four, fur, fair   thigh

Alveolar stops
(tongue tip to alveolar ridge – short sounds)

t	d	n
tea	do	**knee**
two	die	no
tar	day	near
tore	**dough**	
toe	dare	
tie		
tear		
toy		
it	odd	on
eat	**add**	in
ate	aid	earn
oat		

P This page may be photocopied for instructional use only. *Lemon & Lime Library* © R Palmer & A Protopapas 2008

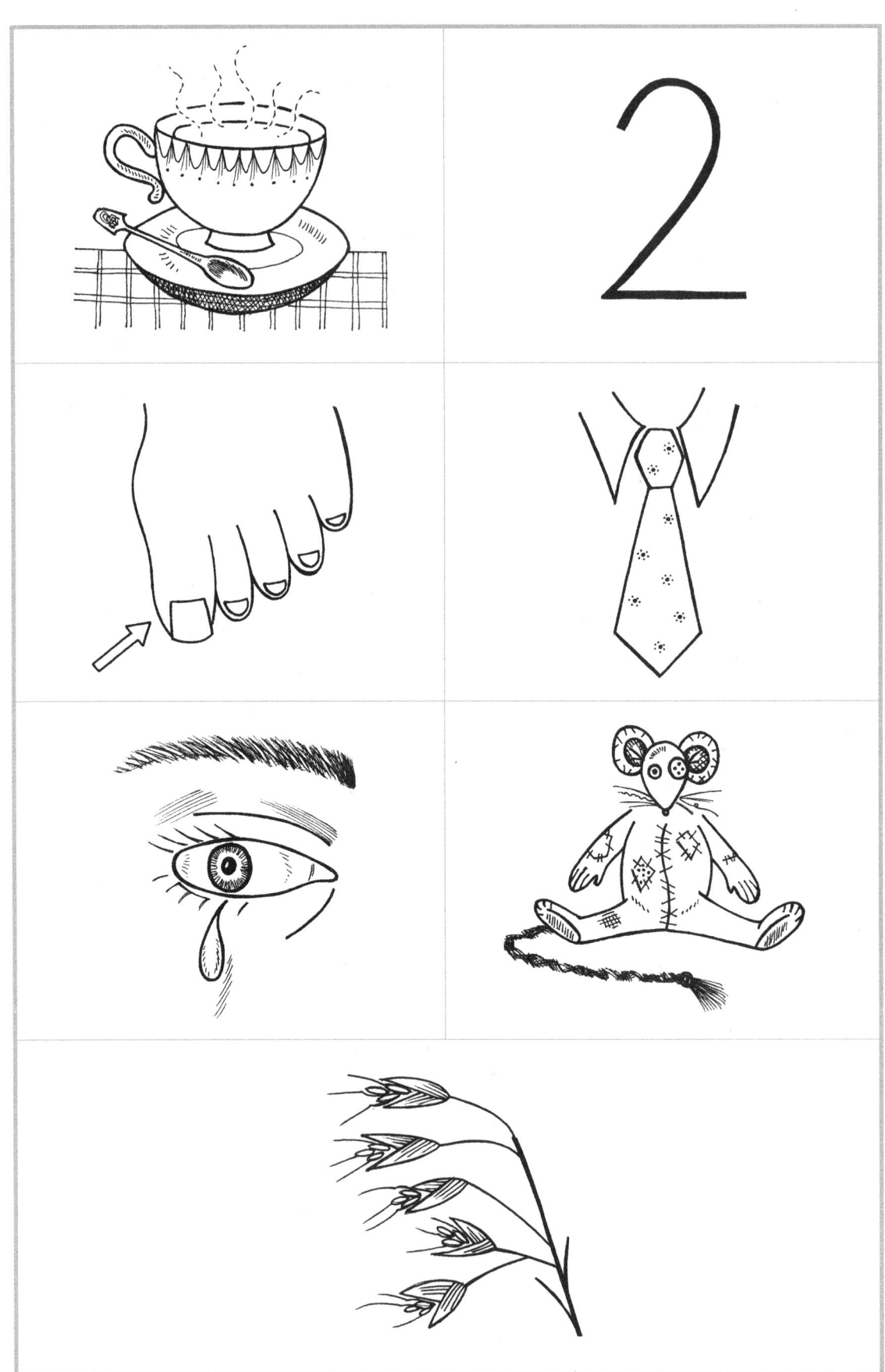

tea, two, toe, tie, tear, toy, oat

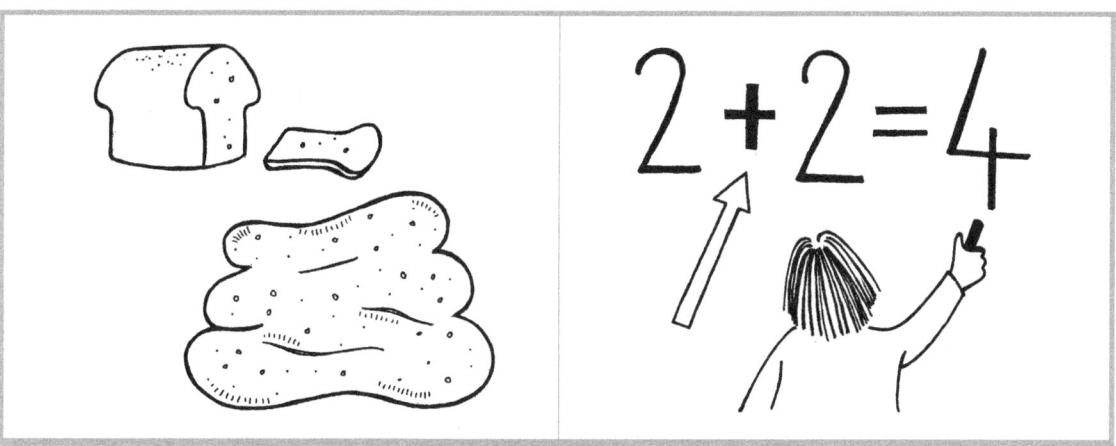

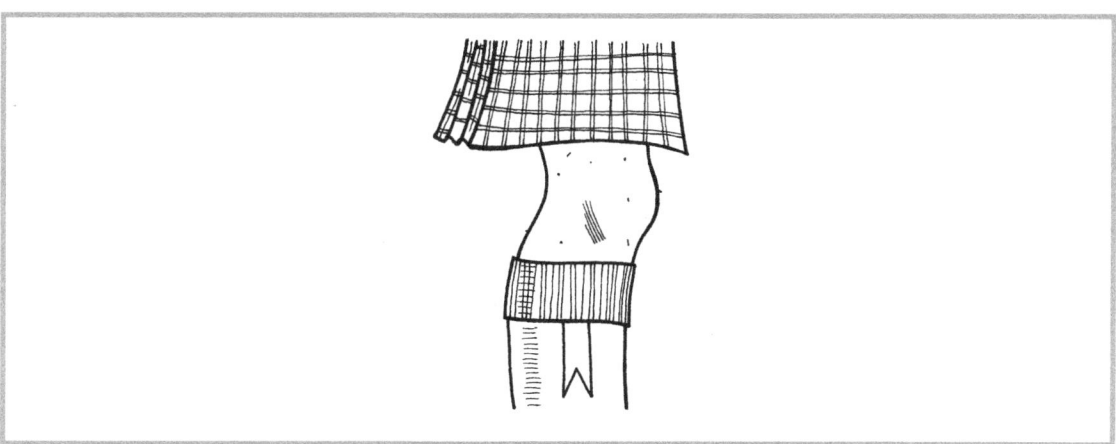

dough, add   knee

Alveolar and post alveolar fricatives
(long sounds with tongue tip on or just behind alveolar ridge)

s	z	sh
saw	**zoo**	she
sue		shore
sir		show
sow		
sigh		
say		
us	is	ash

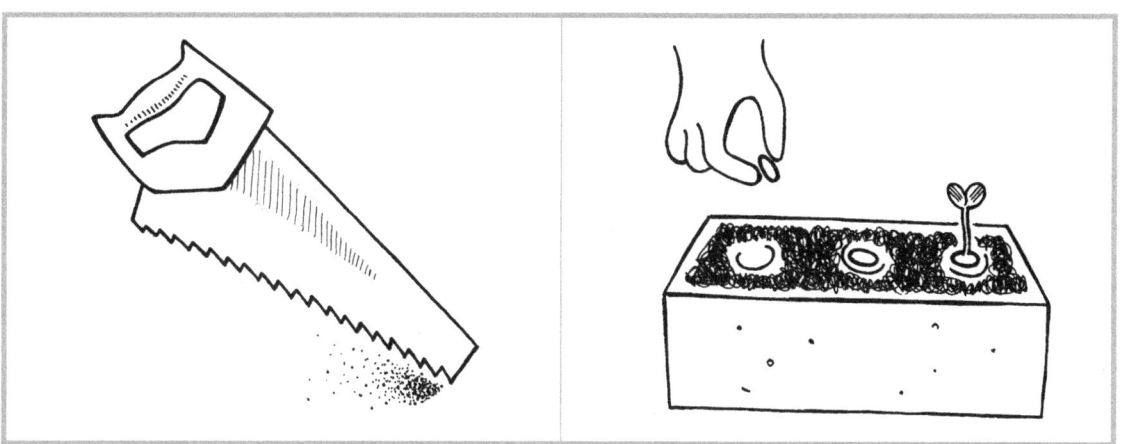

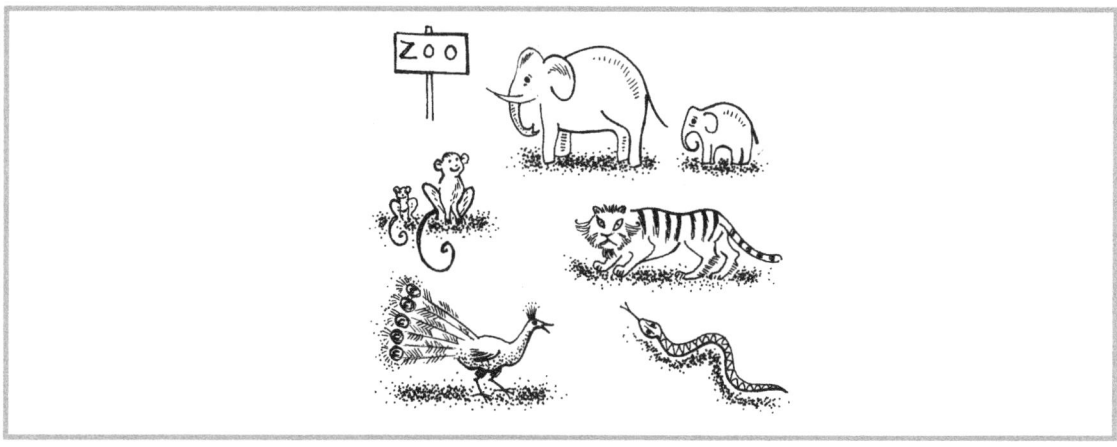

saw, sow   zoo

Post alveolar affricates

ch	j
chew	**jar**
chore	joy
itch	age

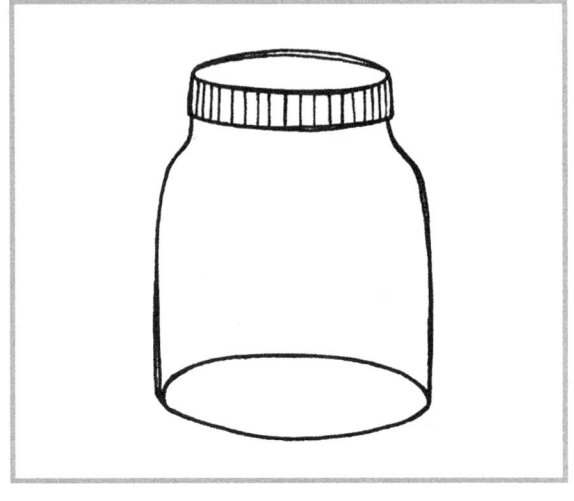

jar

Velars
(back of tongue to palate)

k	g
car	guy
core	go
key	
cow	
care	
coy	
ache	egg

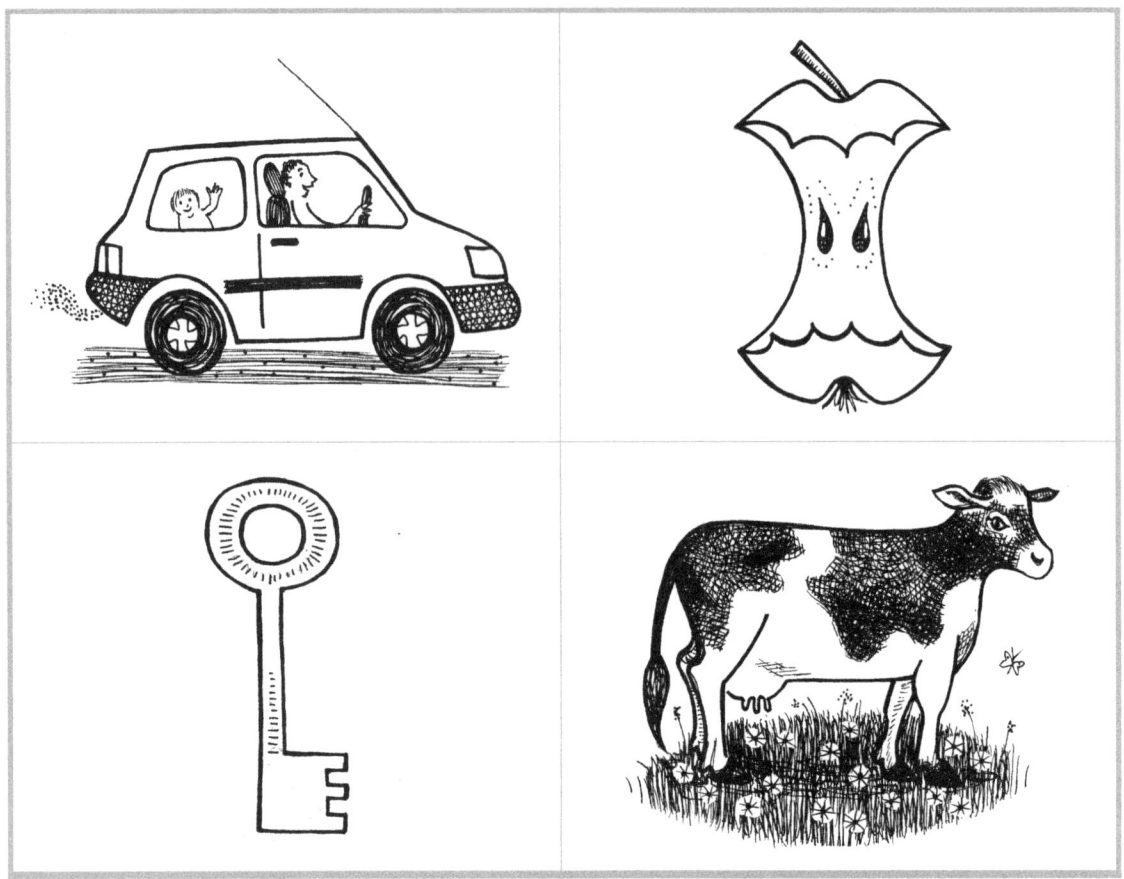

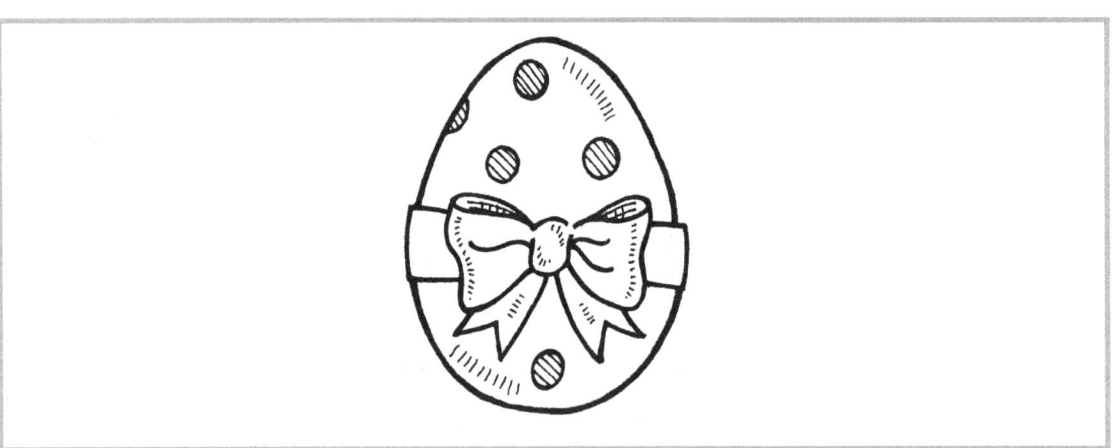

car, core, key, cow   egg

Approximants

l	r	w	j	h
law	raw	wore	your	he
lie	row	we	you	who
low	rare	wear	yeah	her
lay	**ray**	why		**hay**
	rye	weigh		high
ill		wow		hair
all				
earl				
aisle				
ale				

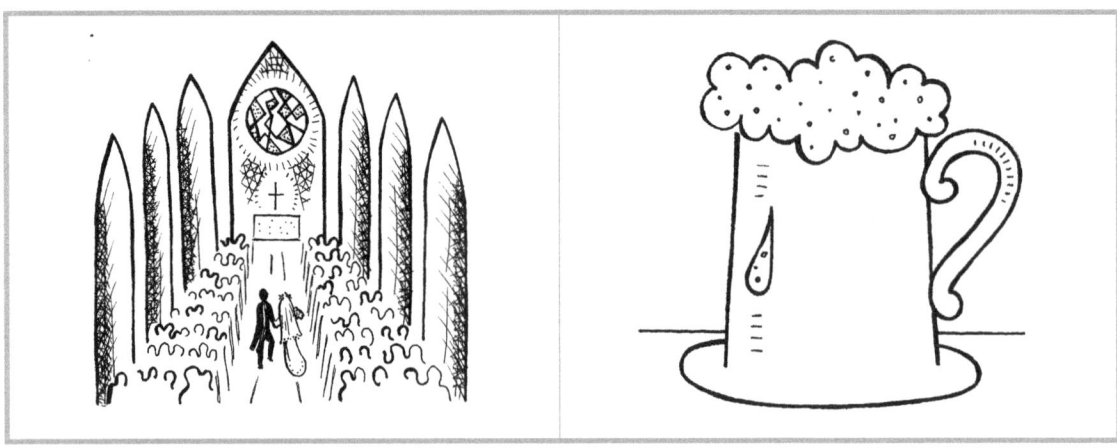

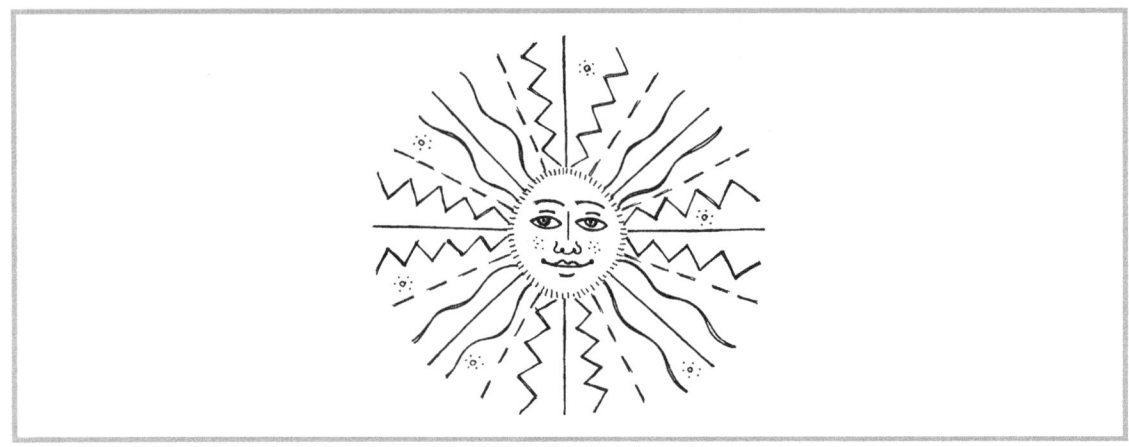

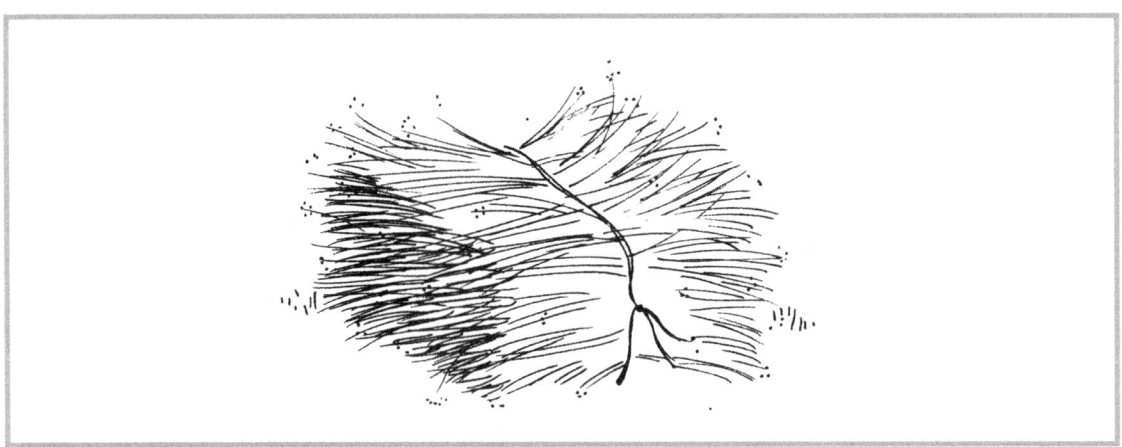

aisle, ale   ray   hay

LEVEL 2 CV and VC words sorted according to vowel

Short vowels

ɪ	e	æ	ʌ	ʊ	ɒ	ə
itch						the
is						
in					on	
it		ash			odd	
if	egg	add	us		off	up
ill						

Long vowels

iː	uː	ɜ	aː	ɔː
pea	boo	fur	pa	poor
bee	moo	sir	baa	bore
me	two	her	ma	more
fee	do		far	four
tea	sue		tar	thaw
knee	chew		jar	tore
she	you		car	saw
key	who			shore
we	zoo			chore
he				core
				law
				raw
				wore
				your
eat		earn		
		earl		all

Diphthongs

eɪ	aɪ	ɔɪ	əʊ	ɑʊ	ɪə	eə	ʊə
pay	pie	boy	mow	cow	beer	pear	
may	bye	joy	foe	wow	tear	bear	
fay	my	toy	toe			fair	
they	thigh		dough			care	
day	tie		no			rare	
say	die		sow			hair	
lay	sigh		show				
ray	guy		go				
weigh	lie		low				
hay	rye	row					
	why						
	high						
ache	aisle		oat				
ate							
aid							
ape							
age							

119

LEVEL 3 Diadochokinetic rate drills repeating the same consonant

LEVEL 3 presents consonants of different phonetic, manner, place and voicing to be repeated several times in consonant – vowel syllables at speed.

Repeat each segment ten times:

papa	baba	mama
fafa	vava	thatha
tata	dada	nana
sasa	zaza	shasha
chacha	jaja	kaka
gaga	wawa	rara
lala	yaya	haha

LEVEL 4 Diadochokinetic rate drills repeating alternating consonants

LEVEL 4 presents CVCV segments in which the consonants differ in place, manner or voicing. These segments are to be repeated several times at speed, thus alternating consonant place, manner or voicing rapidly.

Repeat each segment ten times:

Change in place

Bilabial – alveolar	pata	bada	
Alveolar – velar	taka	daga	kala
Bilabial – velar	paka	baga	

Change in manner

Stop – fricative	tasa	kasha
Nasal – oral	maba	nasa

Change in voicing

Voiced – voiceless	paba	tada	kaga

LEVEL 5 Short words

LEVEL 5 presents lists of words containing each consonant of the English language in word initial, word medial and word final position. Lists of English consonant clusters are also presented. Pictures of imageable words are presented and word lists and pictures can be photocopied for speech practice.

p	123		sh	154	
b	126		Z (as in measure)	157	
m	130		ch	158	
f	133		j	161	
v	136		k	164	
th (as in think)	138		g	168	
th (as in this)	140		l	170	
t	141		r	173	
d	144		w	175	
n	147		y	177	
s	150		h	178	
z	153		ng	180	

Clusters – in word initial position

pl	182		kw	194	
pr	182		gl	197	
bl	184		gr	197	
br	184		sl	199	
fl	187		sm	199	
fr	187		sn	199	
thr	189		sp	201	
tr	190		st	201	
dr	192		sk	201	
kl	194		sw	204	
kr	194				

p

Word initial	Word medial	Word final
pig	depart	**lip**
pink	repair	dip
pet	report	gap
pad	weapon	**map**
pan	**happy**	chop
past	topic	top
pot	copy	
push	**supper**	
pool	**people**	heap
palm	**pupil**	loop
part		**soup**
park		
page	open	escape
pain		hope
paint		pope
pale		
point		

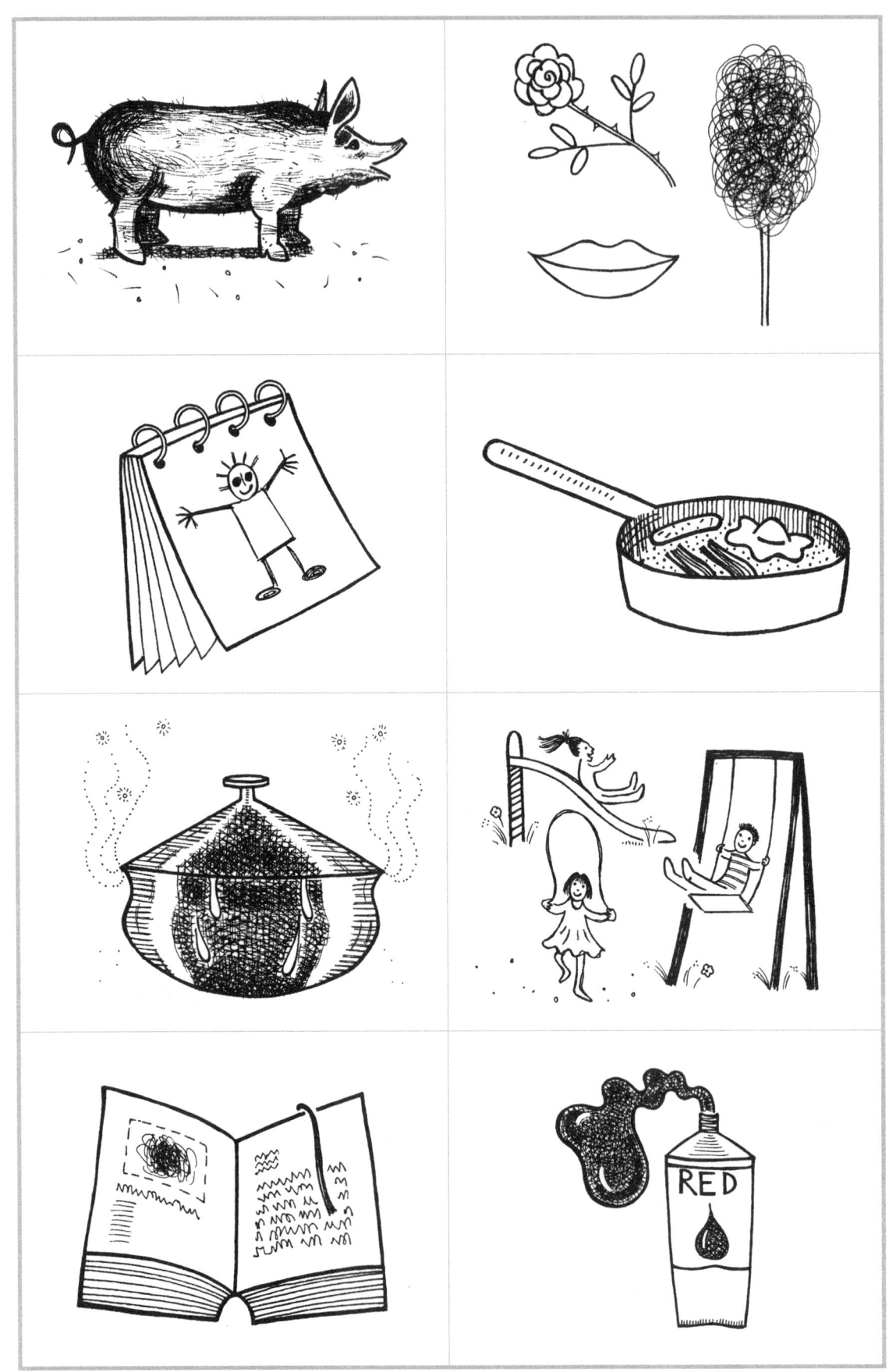

pig, pink, pad, pan, pot, park, page, paint

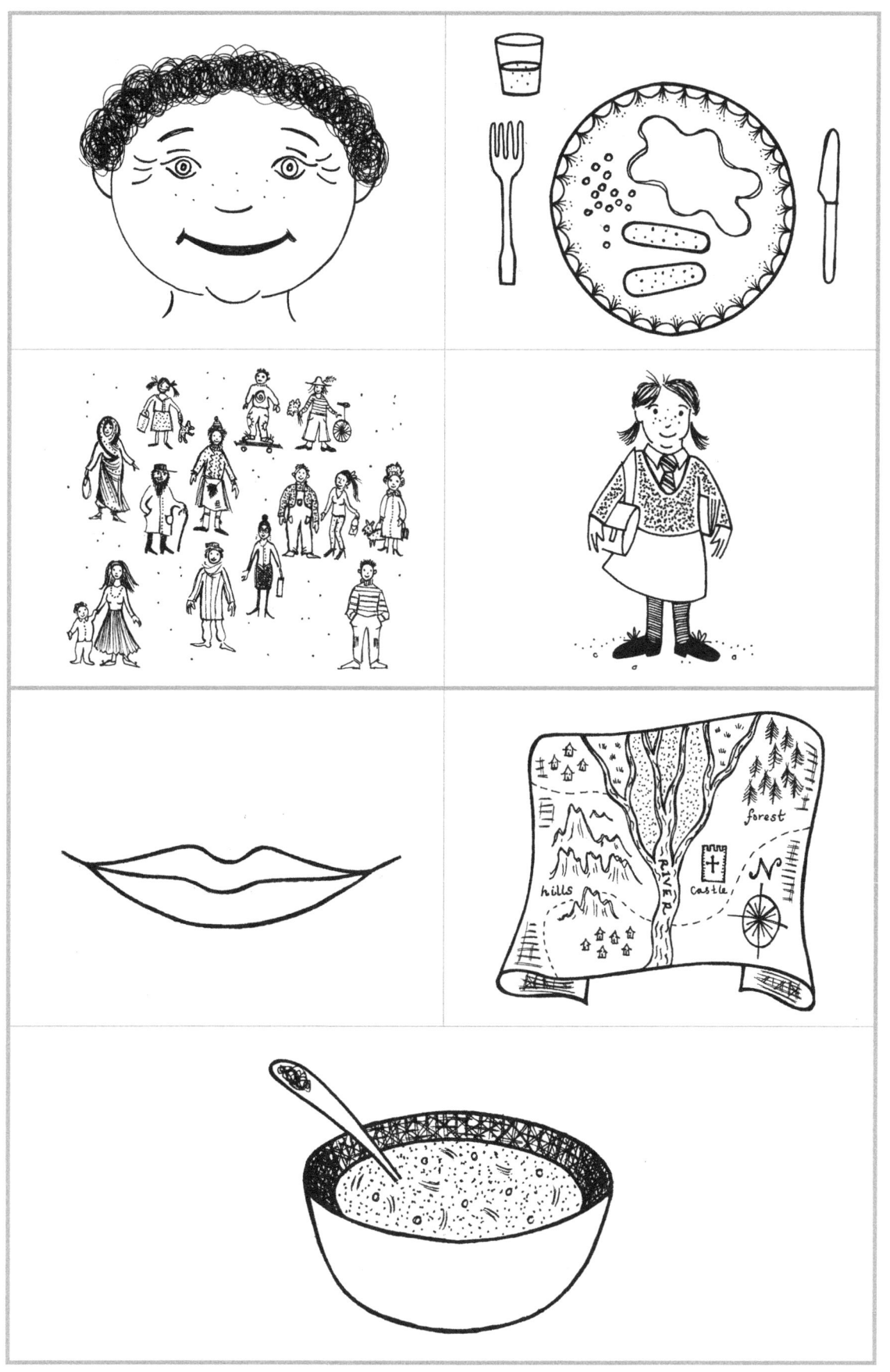

happy, supper, people, pupil   lip, map, soup

Word initial	Word medial	Word final
big	debate	**rib**
bed	cabin	lab
bath	**rabbit**	**cab**
back	habit	grab
bus	**robin**	
	rubbish	
bean		
bird	verbal	
barn		
ball		
bite	**Bible**	
bowl	mobile	

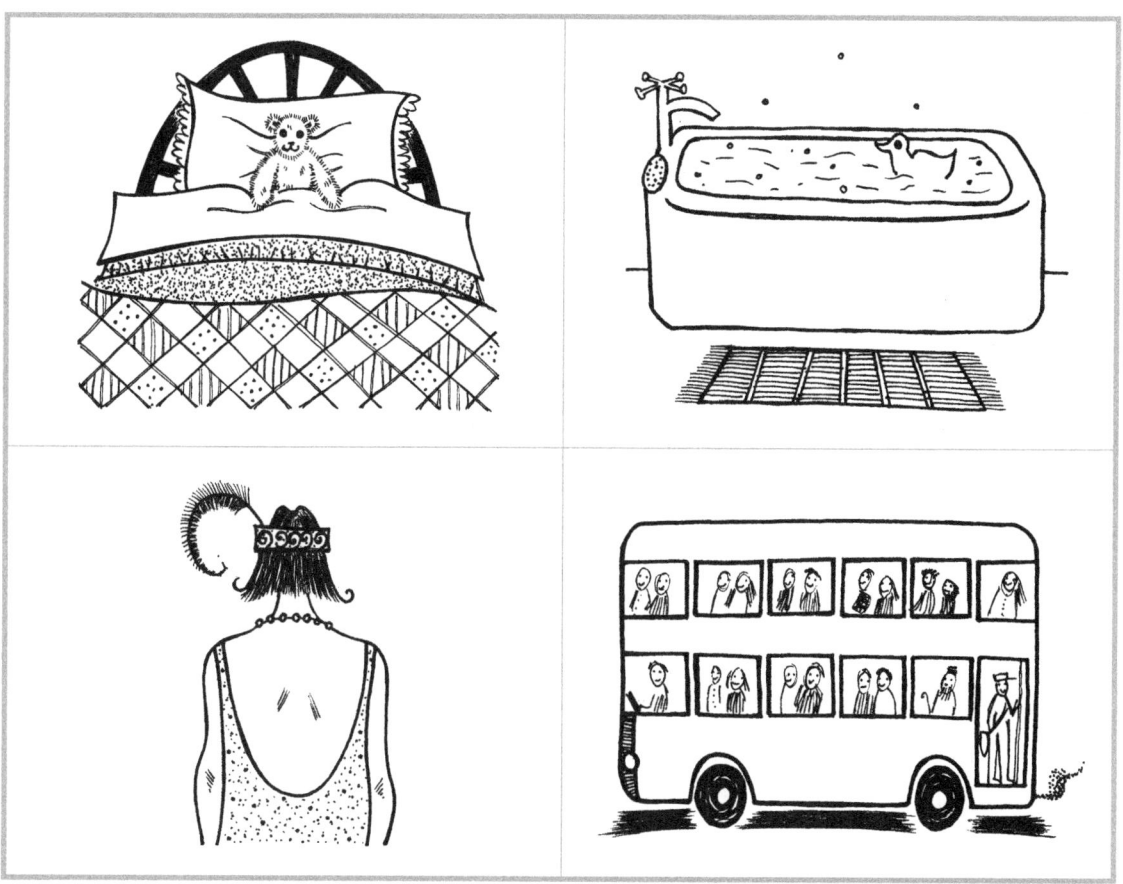

bed, bath, back, bus

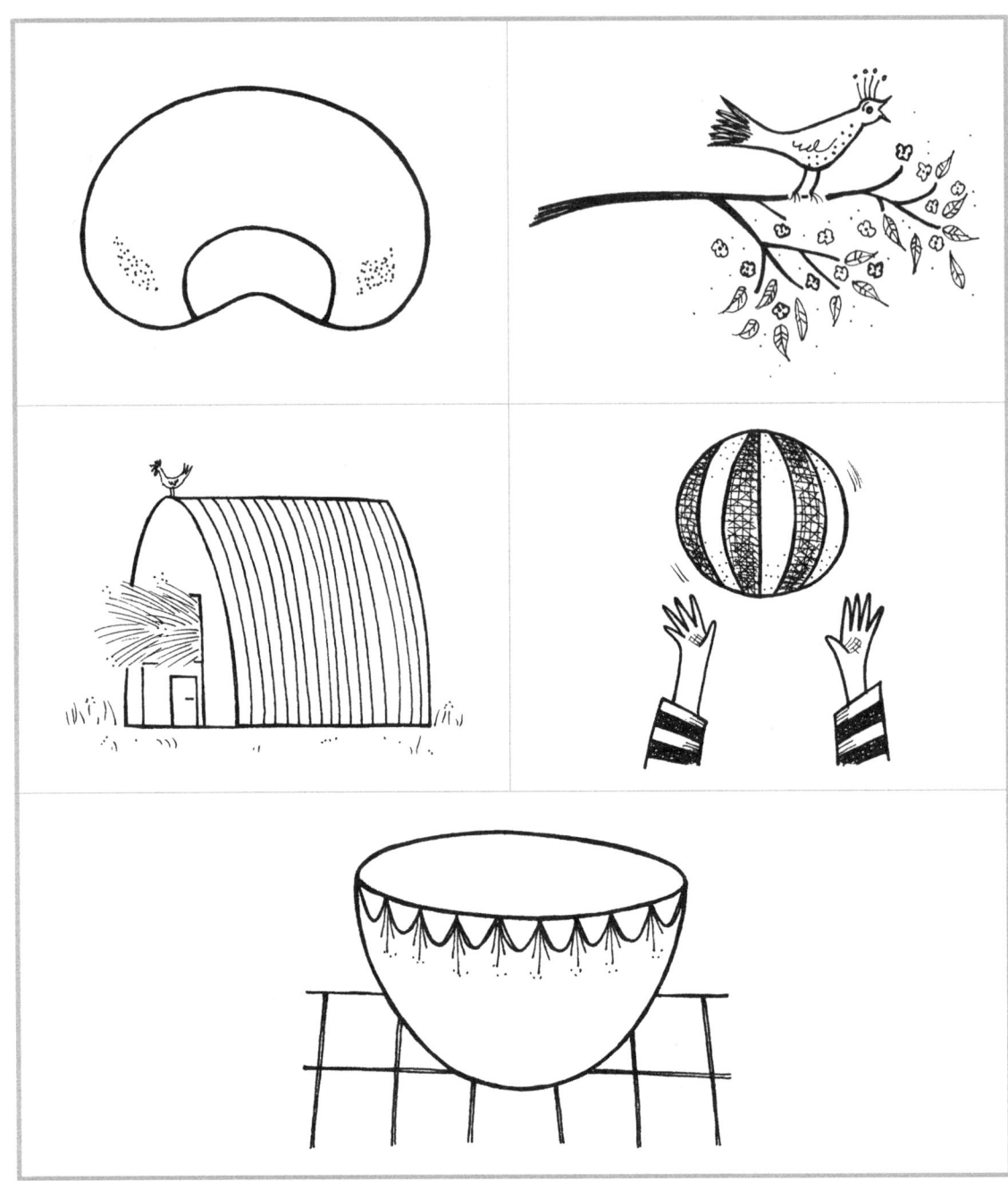

bean, bird, barn, ball, bowl

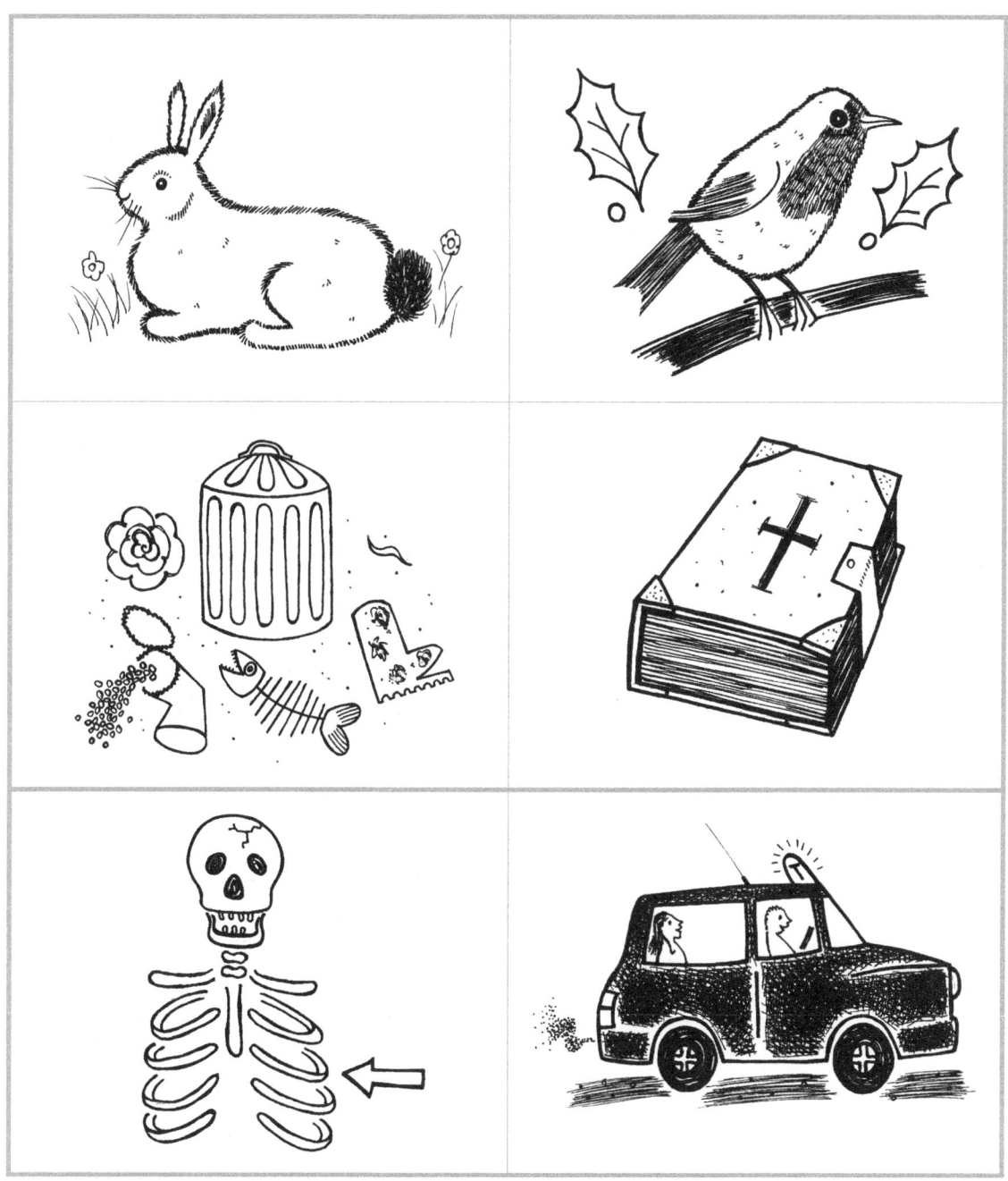

rabbit, robin, rubbish, Bible   rib, cab

m

Word initial	Word medial	Word final
miss	damage	**arm**
mess	common	aim
mad	**mummy**	
mug	**woman**	come
meat	human	team
mood	charming	boom
March	**farmer**	calm
		harm
maid	famous	**farm**
might	timing	charm
meal		
		game

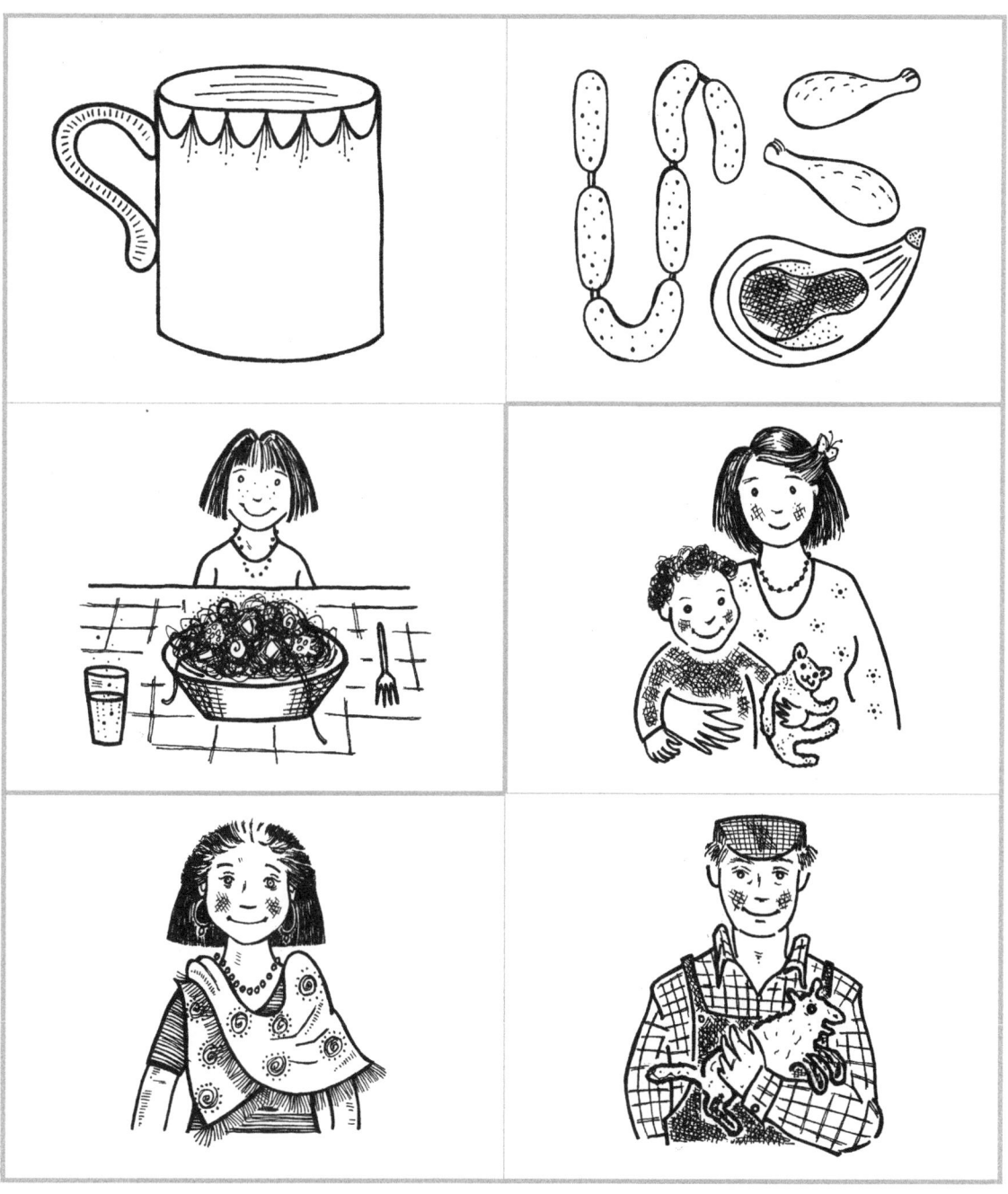

mug, meat, meal   mummy, woman, farmer

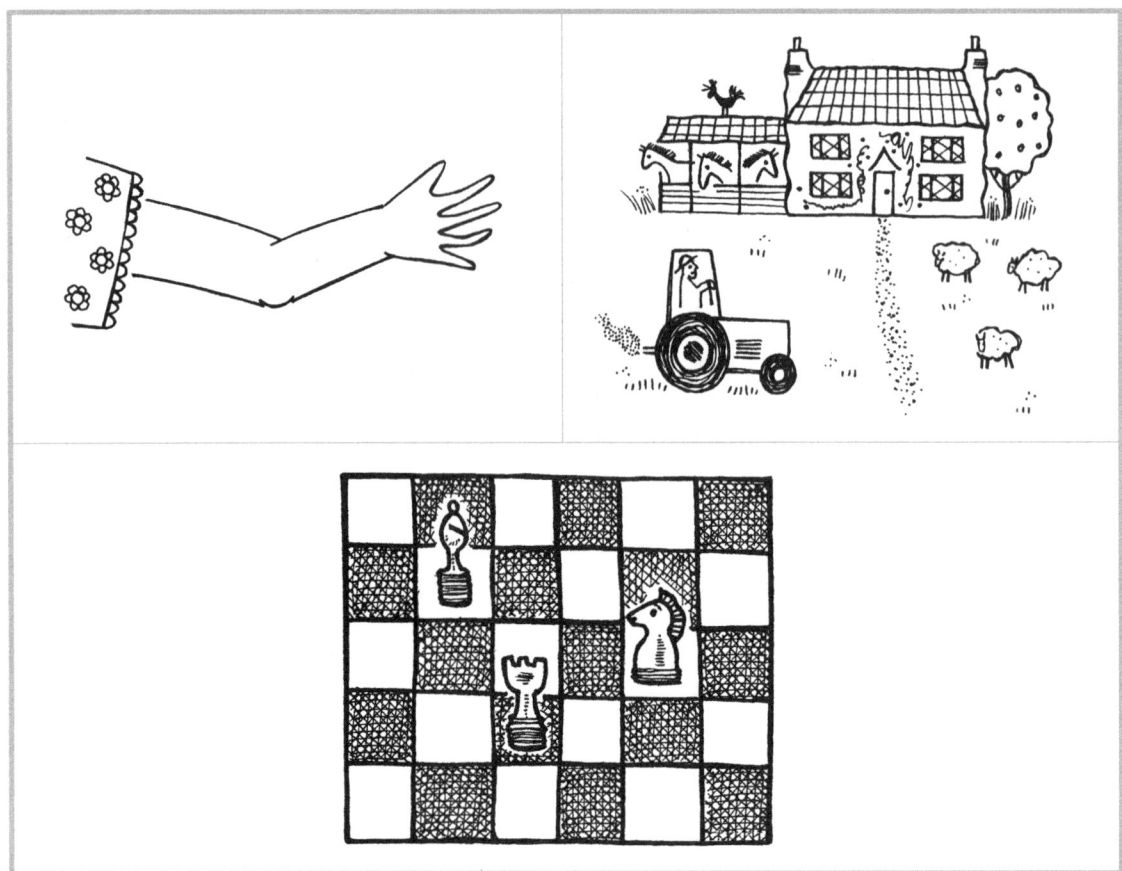

arm, farm, game

f

Word initial	Word medial	Word final
fog	**office**	off
	offer	
food	affair	deaf
force	effort	
ford		**chief**
fall	differ	**leaf**
	define	**roof**
face	before	**calf**
fate	refer	**half**
fair	suffer	
folk		life
fight		

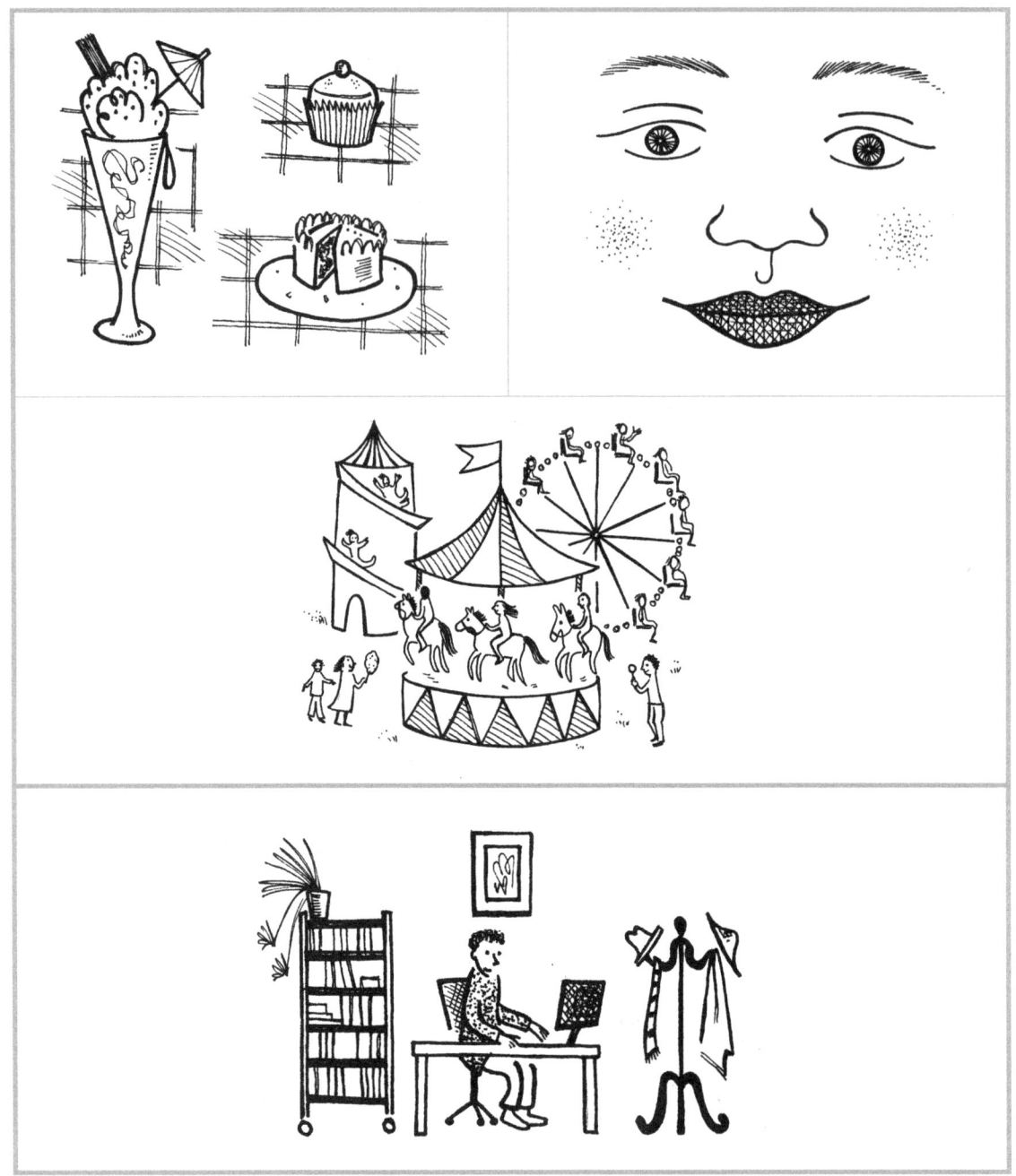

food, face, fair   office

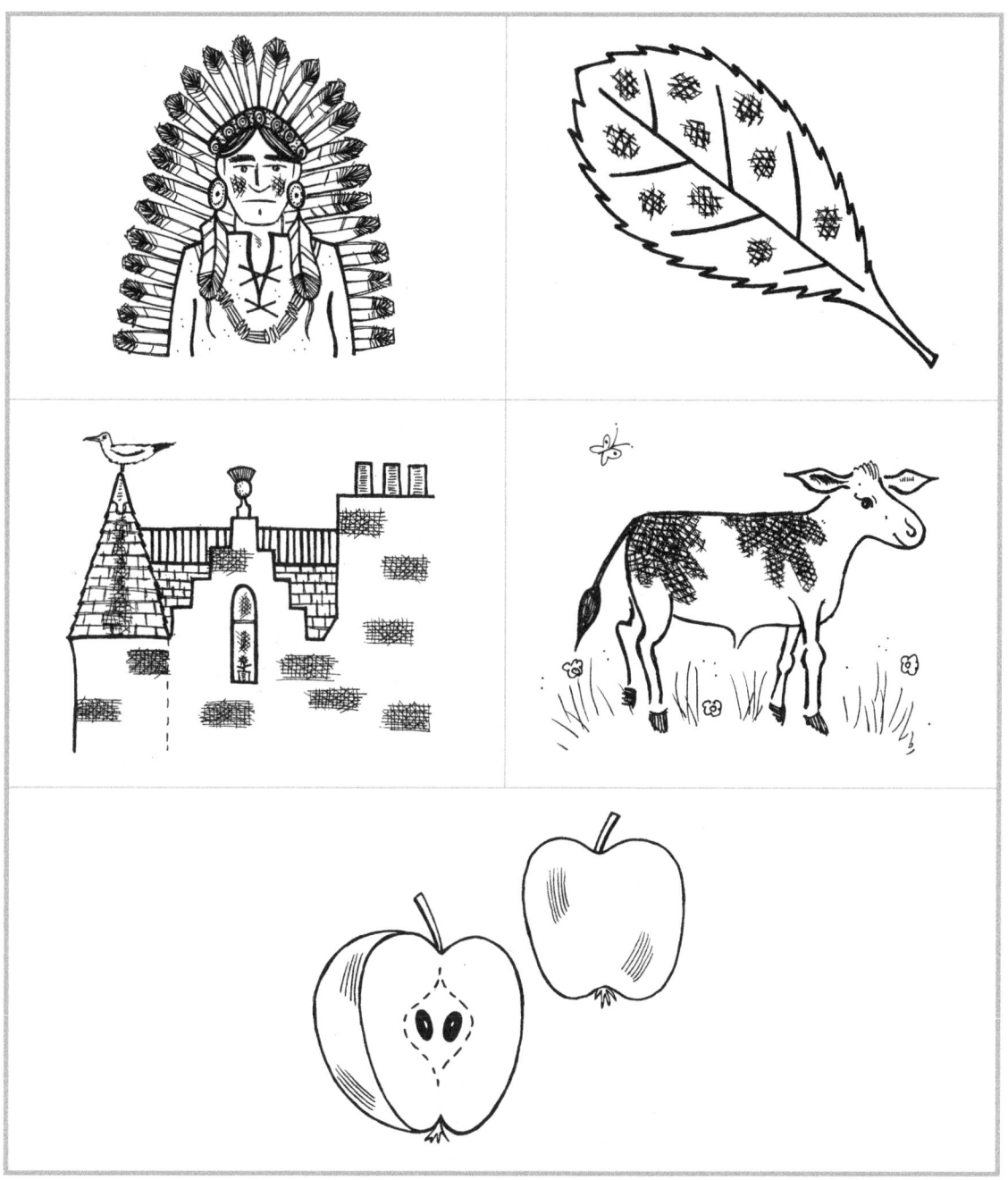

chief, leaf, roof, calf, half

Word initial	Word medial	Word final
villa	evil	of
Venice		
valid	heaven	give
	Devon	have
verse	devise	
	civil	leave
vein	**divide**	nerve
vague	**cover**	serve
voice	servant	
vote		**cave**
view	favour	

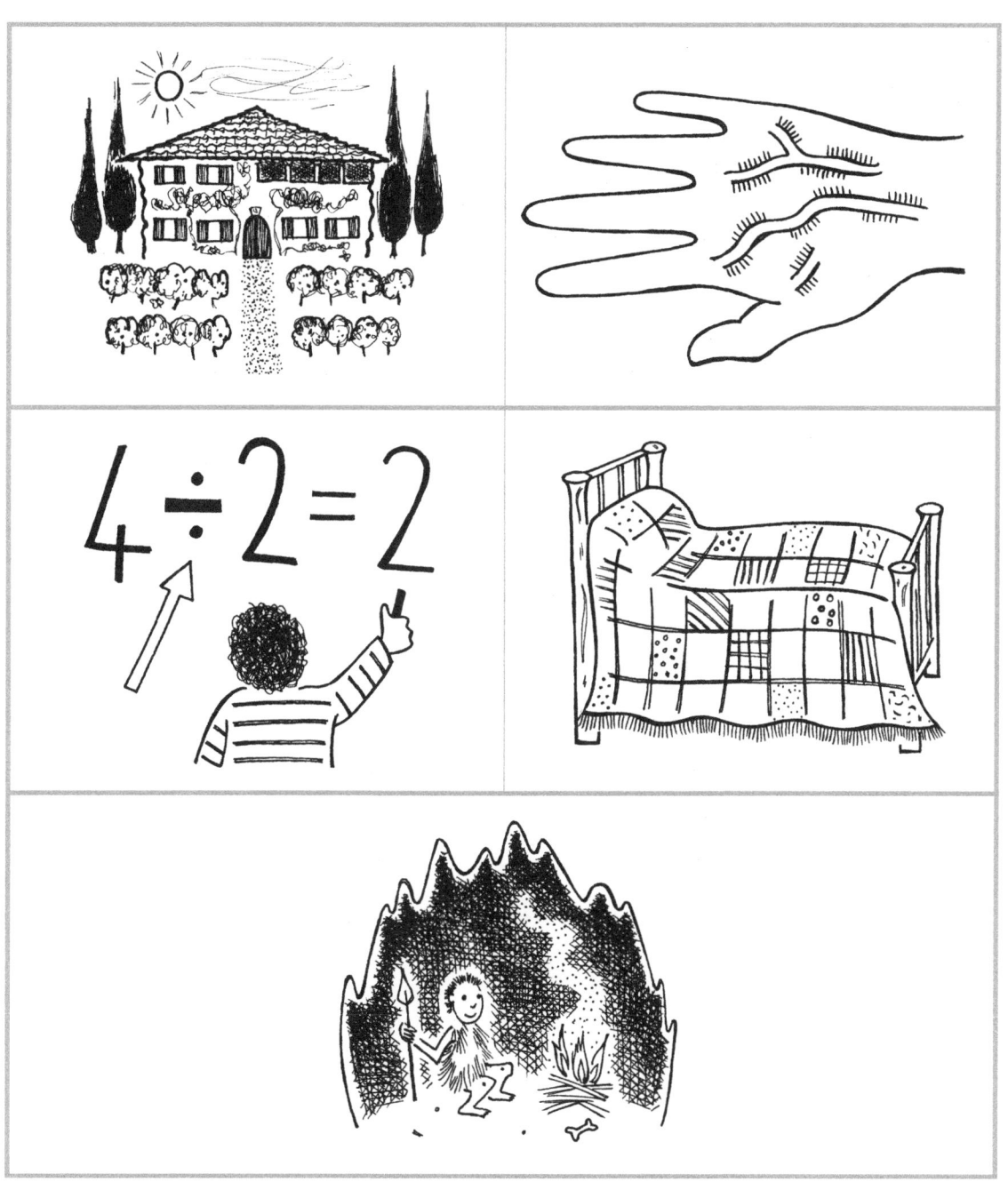

villa, vein   divide, cover   cave

th *(as in think)*

Word initial	Word medial	Word final
thick	author	earth
thin		
thank	gothic	breath
thumb	nothing	myth
		bath
theme		
third		birth
thirty	youth	
theory		**south**
		both

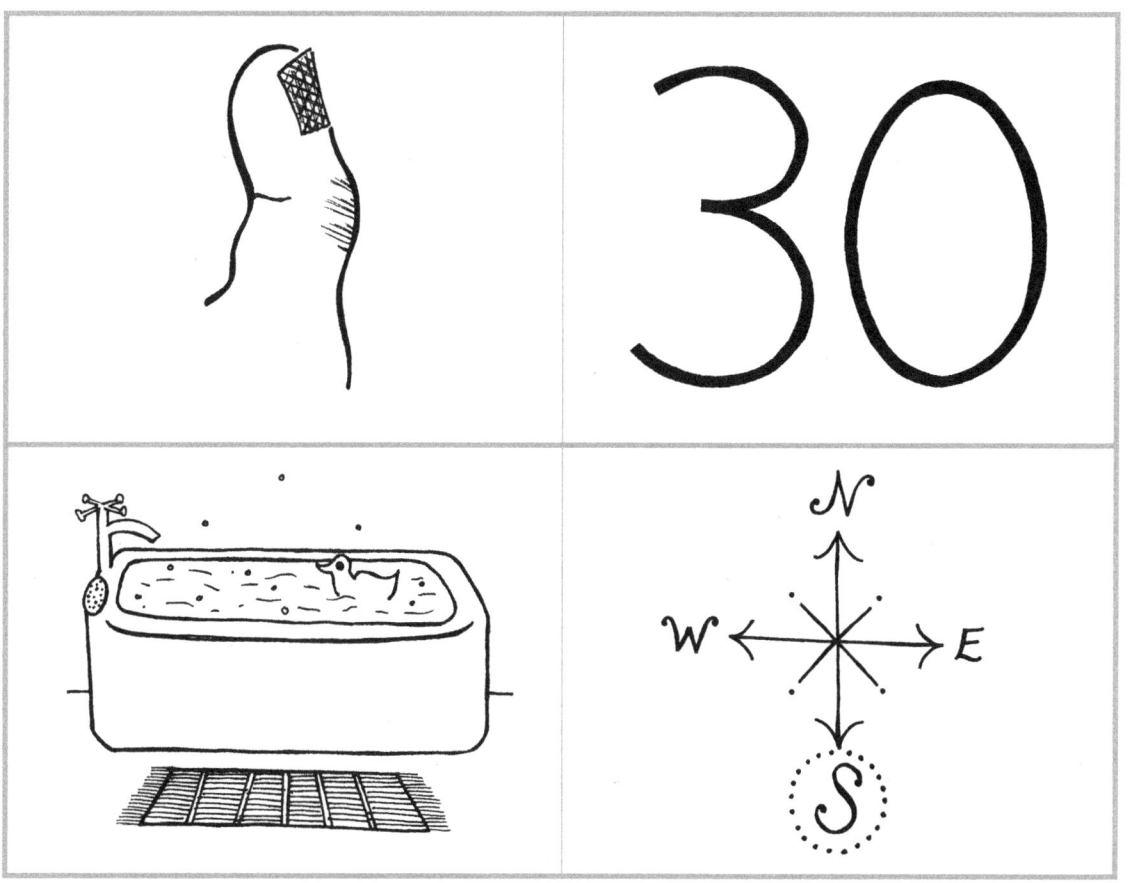

thumb, thirty   bath, south

th *(as in this)*

Word initial	Word medial	Word final
then	either	breathe
than		smooth
thus	**leather**	
	weather	
there	gather	
they	bother	
thou		
though	worthy	
those	further	

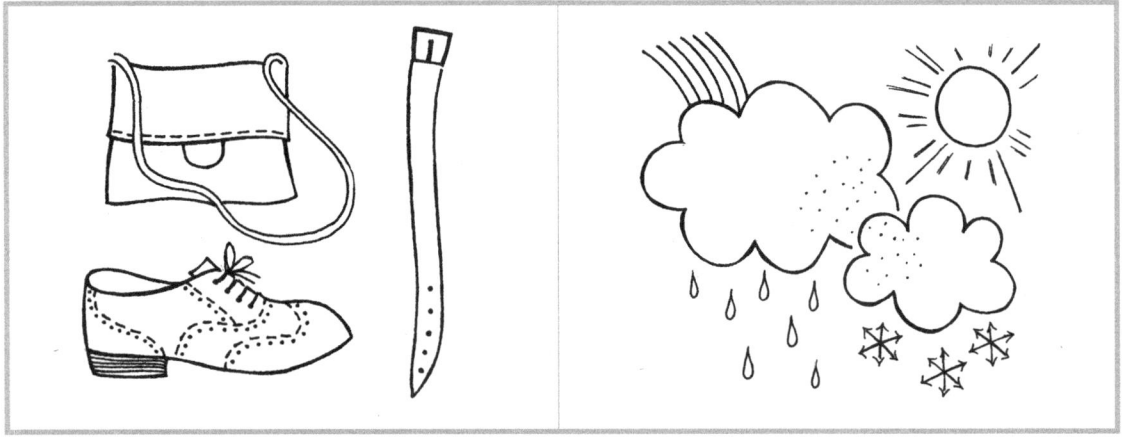

leather, weather

Word initial	Word medial	Word final
tip	attack	bet
tin		**cat**
tap	**sitting**	**bat**
tongue	**cutting**	
	butter	late
teach		**date**
	detail	bite
told	dirty	**note**
tide	daughter	doubt
time		
tail	writing	
	beauty	

141

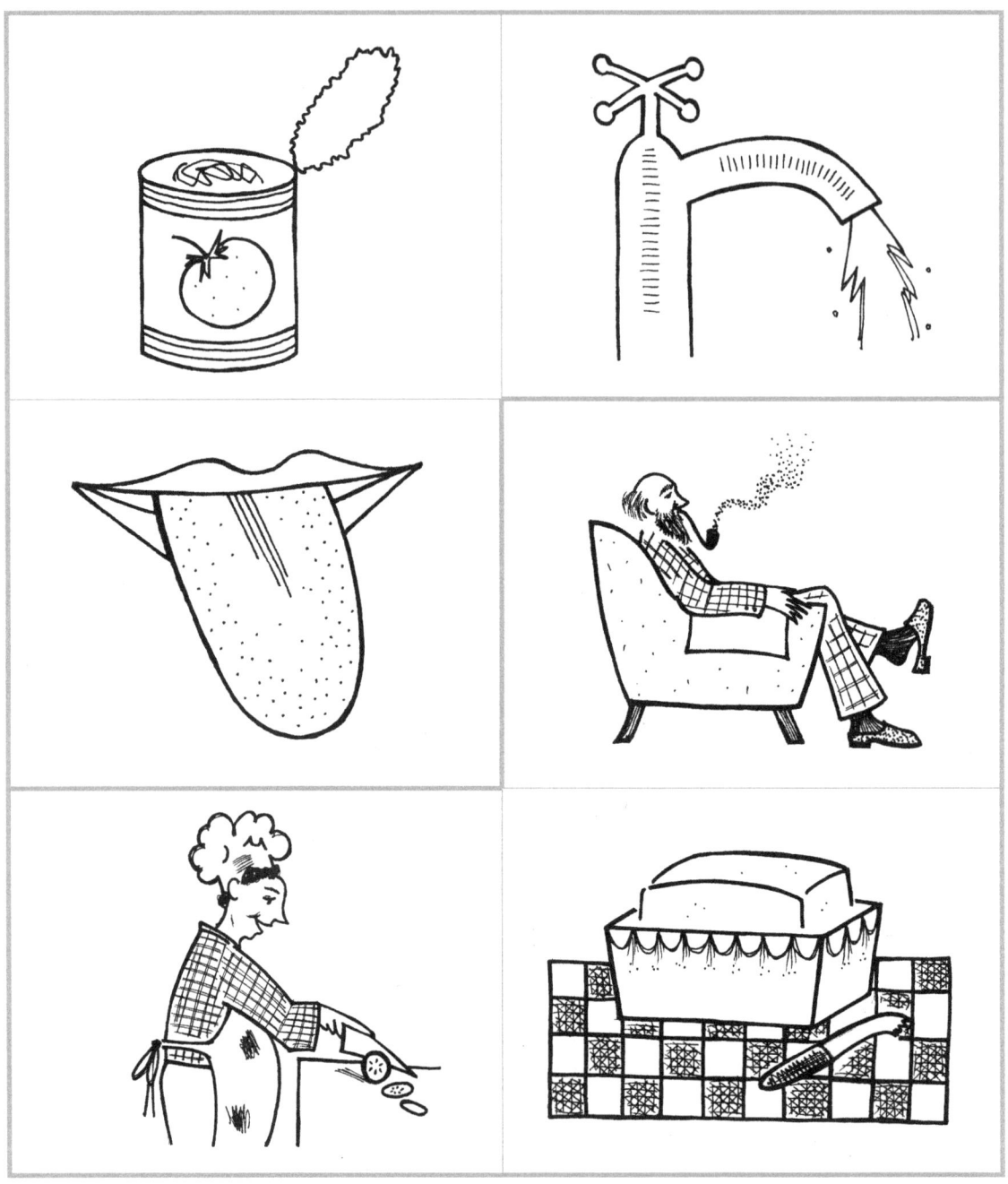

tin, tap, tongue   sitting, cutting, butter

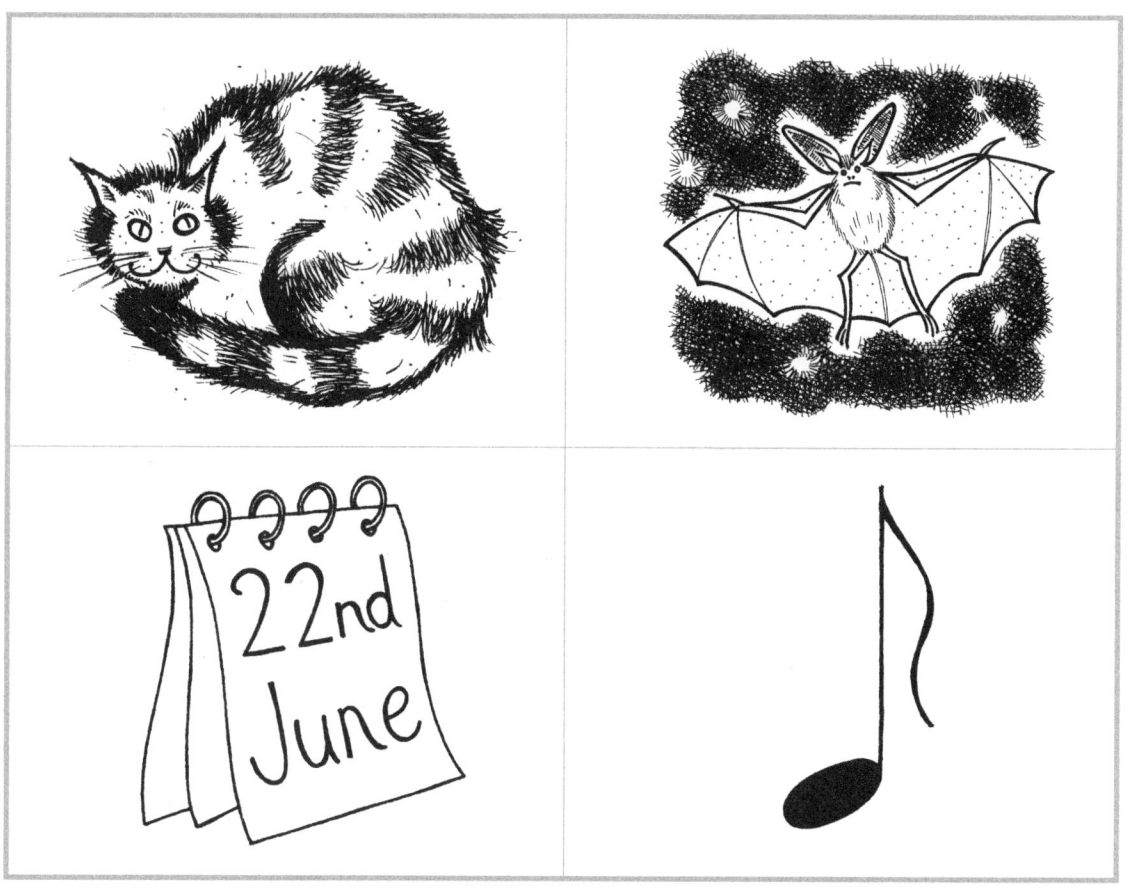

cat, bat, date, note

d

Word initial	Word medial	Word final
dish	order	**bed**
deaf	adding	sad
dad		god
dock	**medal**	
duck	widow	feed
	hidden	**food**
deep	daddy	**sword**
dark	**ladder**	hard
dirt	sudden	
dawn		load
	reading	code
date	pardon	side
doubt	**garden**	

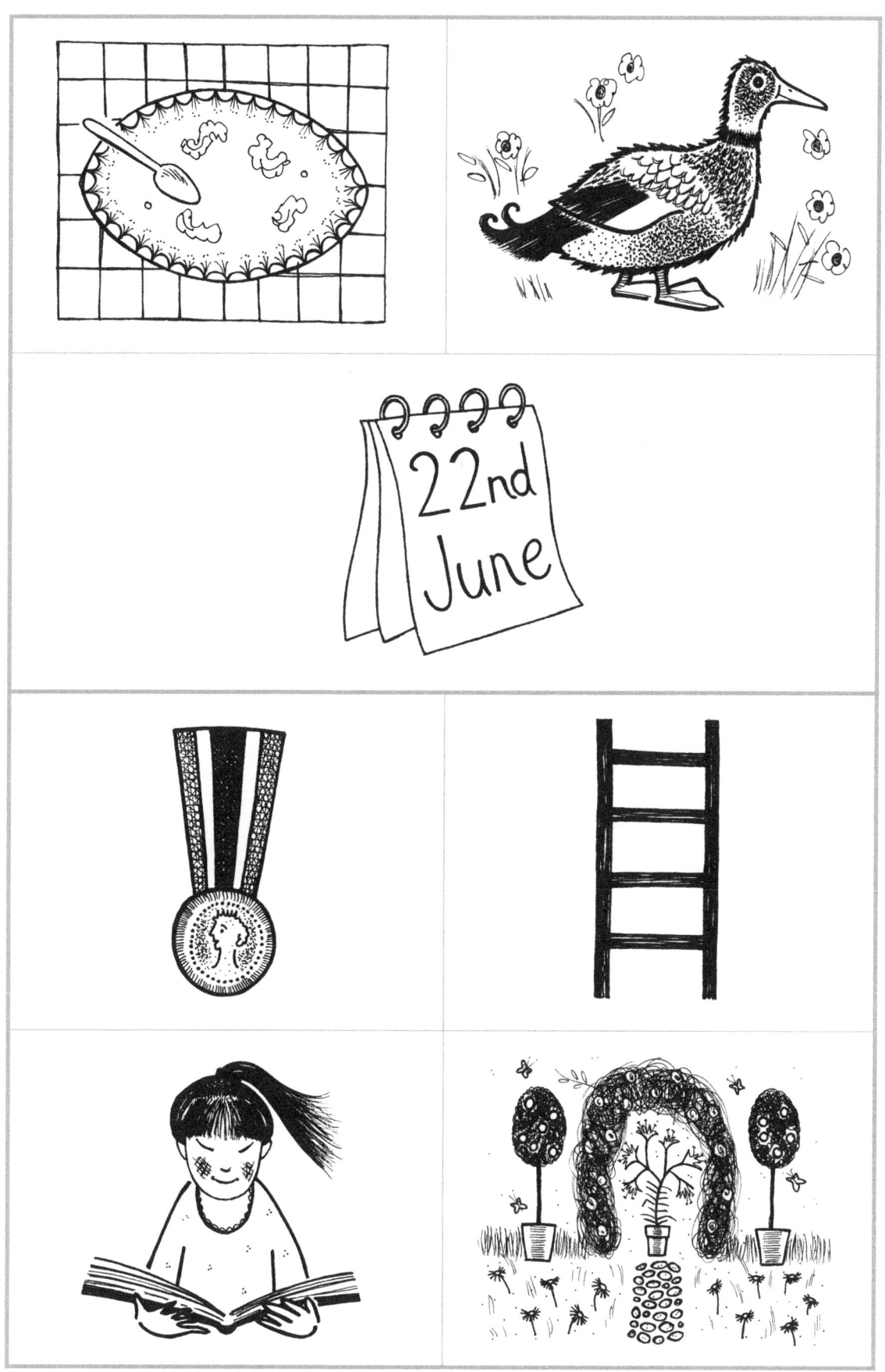

dish, duck, date   medal, ladder, reading, garden

145

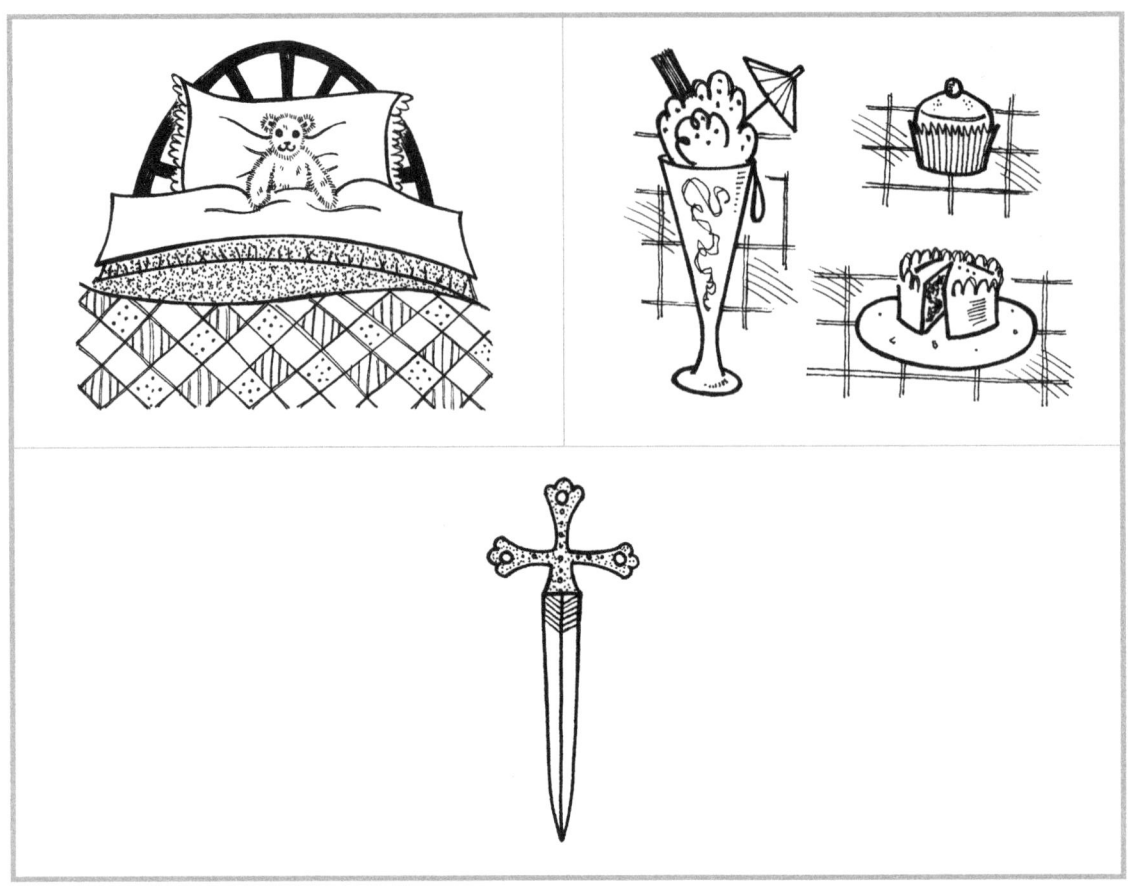

bed, food, sword

Word initial	Word medial	Word final
neck	**dinner**	**tin**
nut	finish	then
	menu	**pan**
neat	Venice	
nerve	manage	**bean**
nurse	funny	barn
north	**honey**	
	running	pain
name	**sunny**	**vein**
nice		shine
note		join

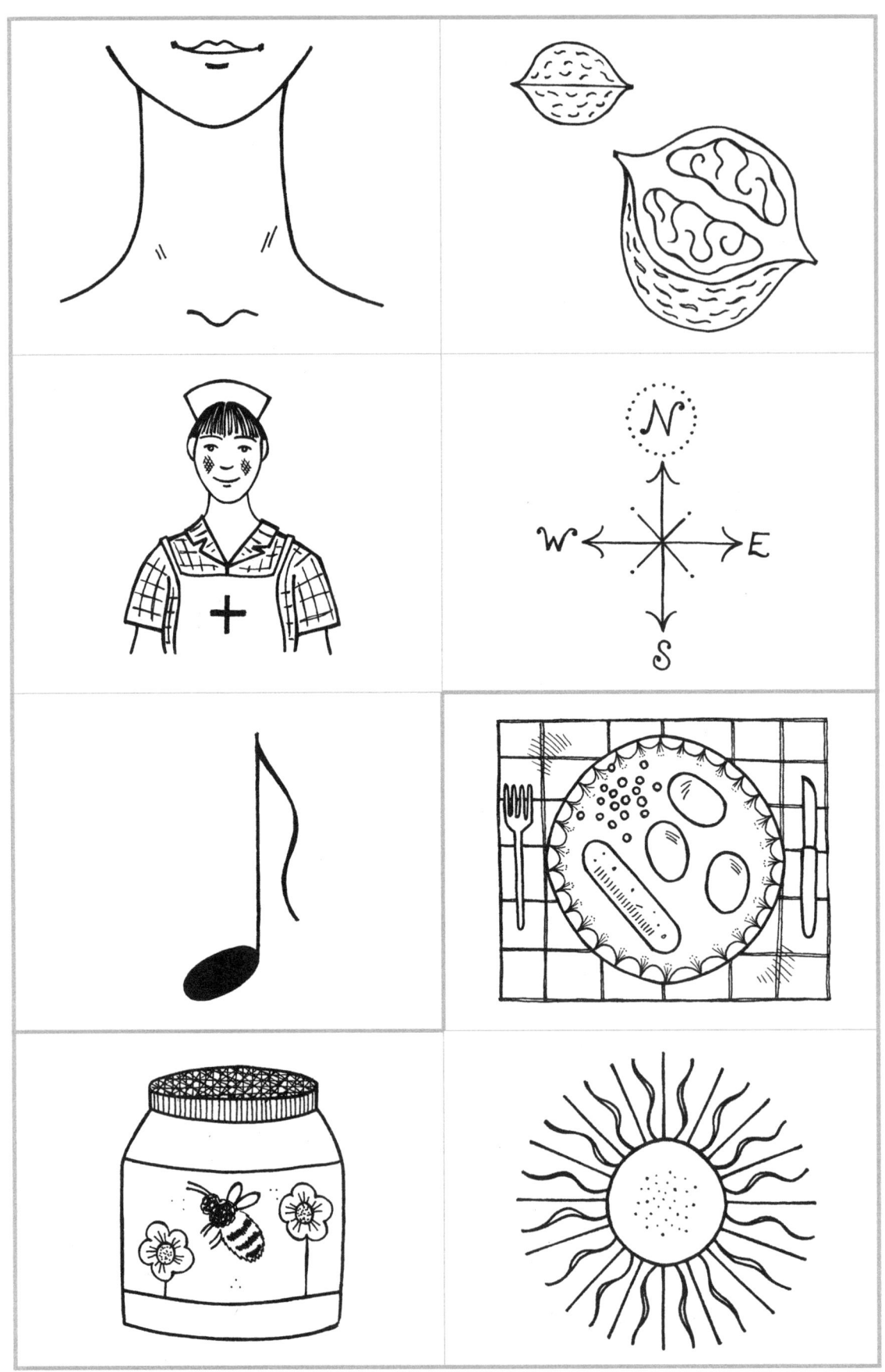

neck, nut, nurse, north, note   dinner, honey, sunny

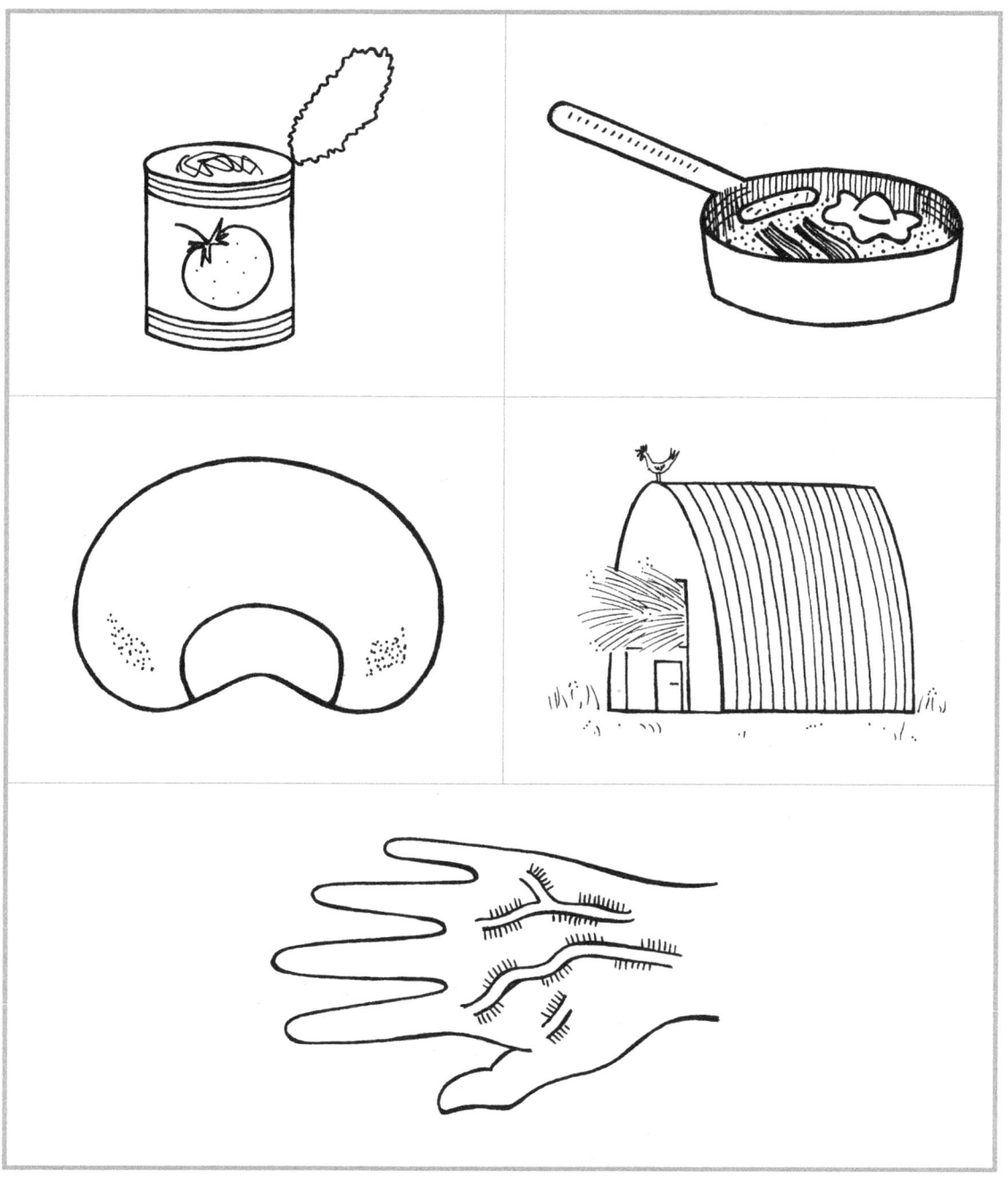

tin, pan, bean, barn, vein

Word initial	Word medial	Word final
set	acid	gas
sad		**bus**
sock	beside	
	decide	verse
soup	**message**	force
seat	lesson	**juice**
sauce		
	horses	**face**
safe	mercy	**lace**
side		choice
soap	**faces**	voice
seal	**basin**	

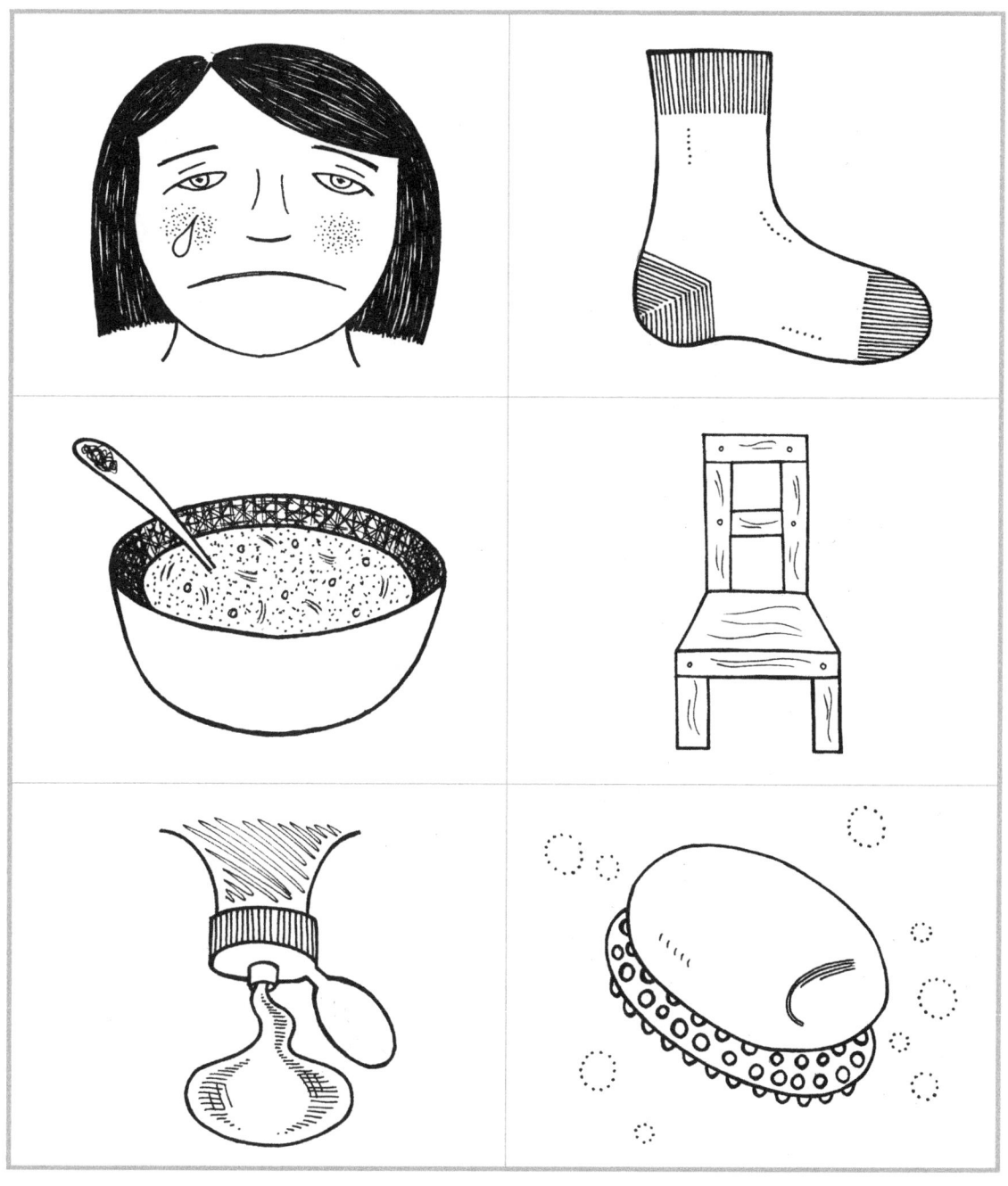

sad, sock, soup, seat, sauce, soap

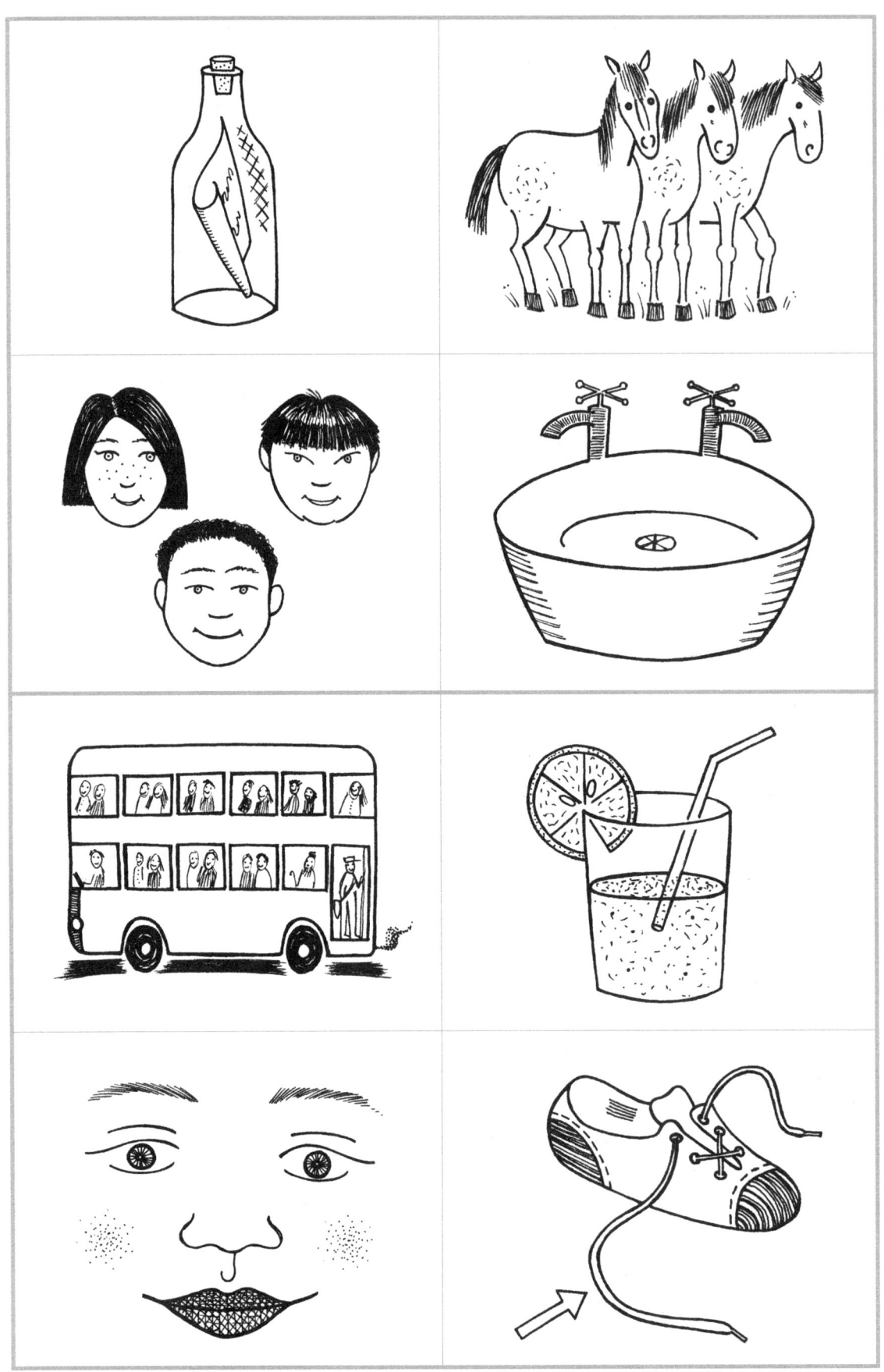

message, horses, faces, basin   bus, juice, face, lace

Word initial	Word medial	Word final
zero	resign	jazz
	design	
	visit	choose
	present	
	busy	gaze
		wise
	reason	those
		rose
	noisy	
	trousers	

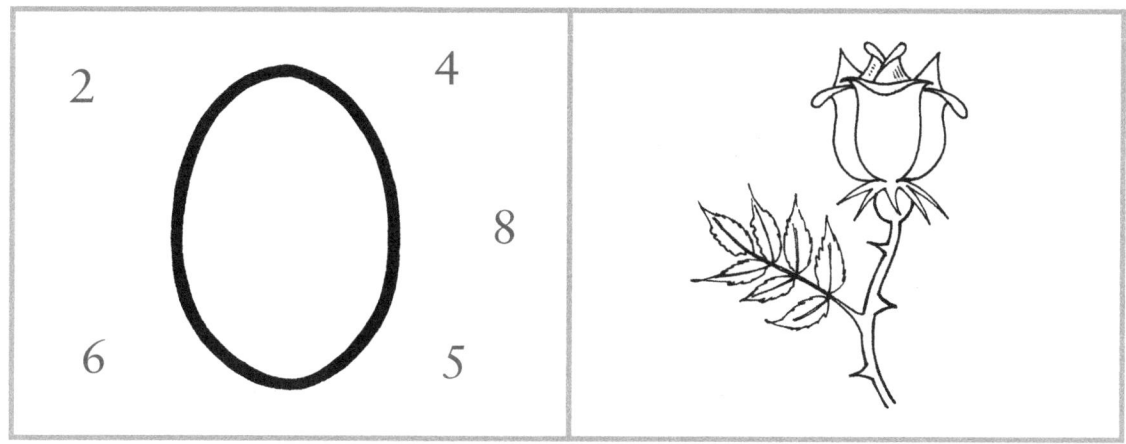

zero   rose

Word initial	Word medial	Word final
shed	issue	wish
ship	ocean	**dish**
shop		**cash**
shut	bishop	**crash**
	dishes	rush
short	**fishing**	**push**
shoot	**tissue**	**bush**
shirt	session	**wash**
sheep	fashion	
sharp	**pushing**	harsh
shade	portion	
share		
shout	nation	
shine		

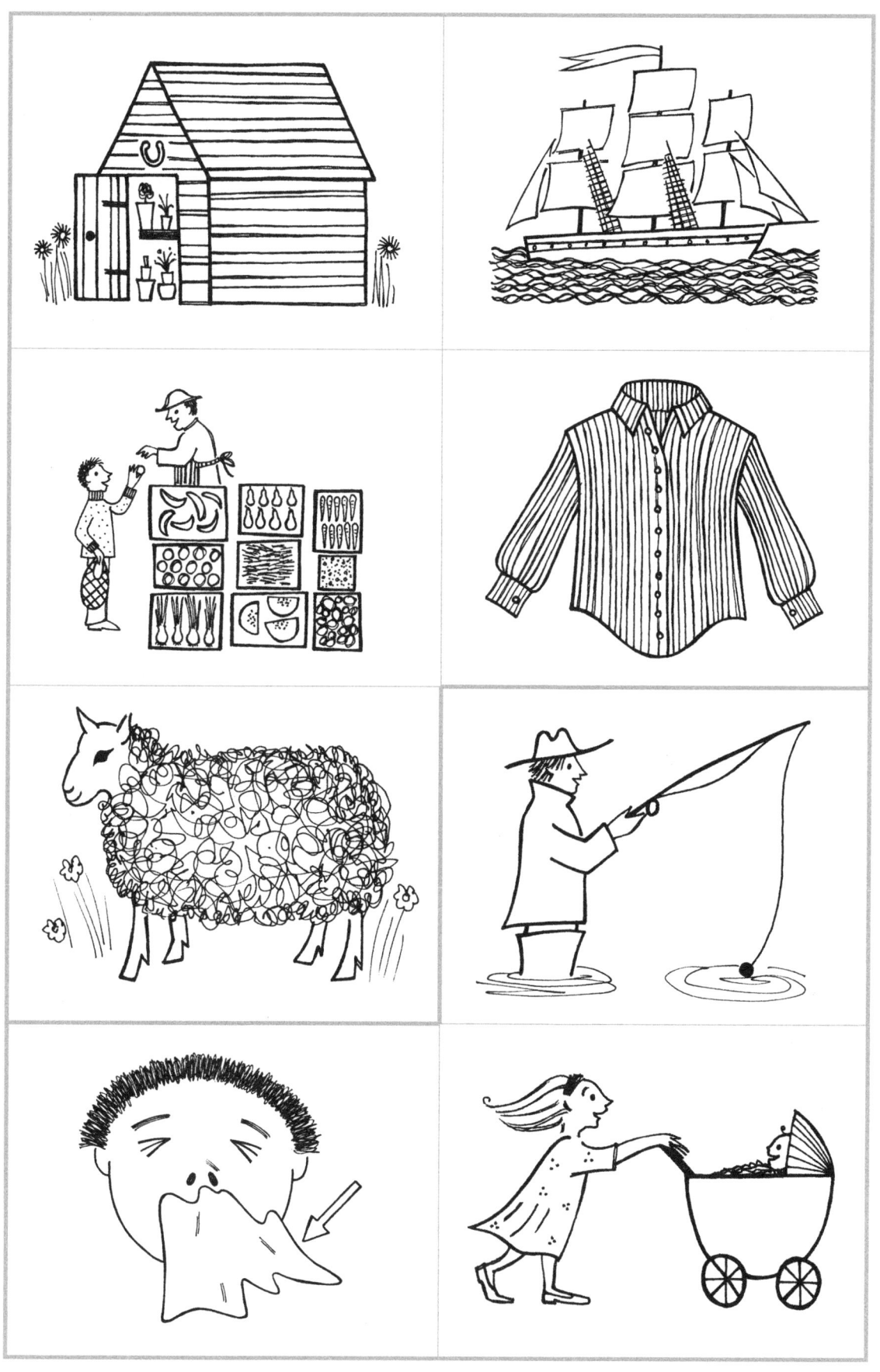

shed, ship, shop, shirt, sheep   fishing, tissue, pushing

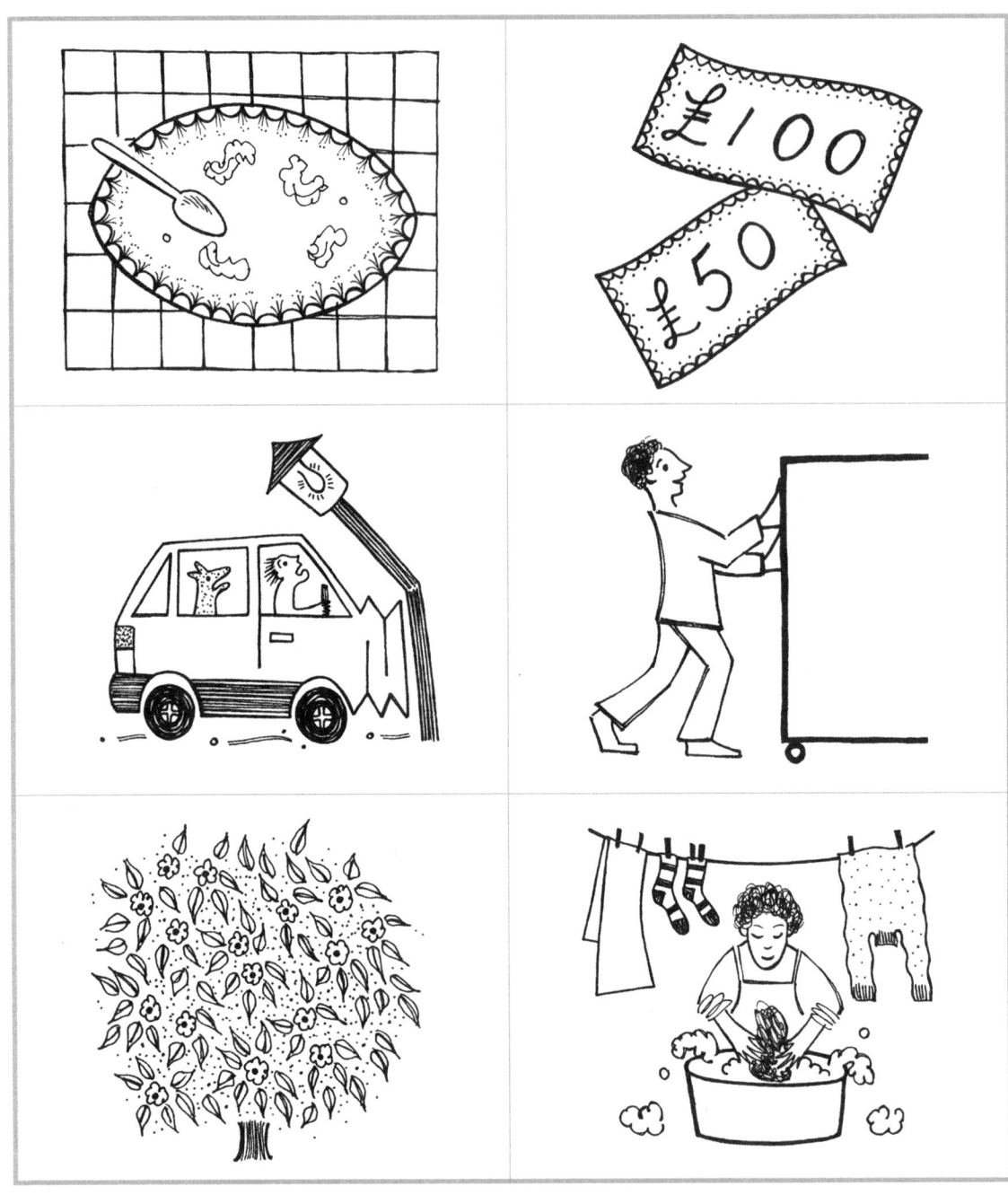

dish, cash, crash, push, bush, wash

Z (as in measure)

Word initial	Word medial	Word final
	casual	
	version	

157

Word initial	Word medial	Word final
chin	kitchen	patch
check	stretching	match
chap	watching	catch
chop		much
	feature	watch
cheep	teacher	
chart	fortune	teach
choose	purchase	reach
		march
chain	nature	launch
choice	future	

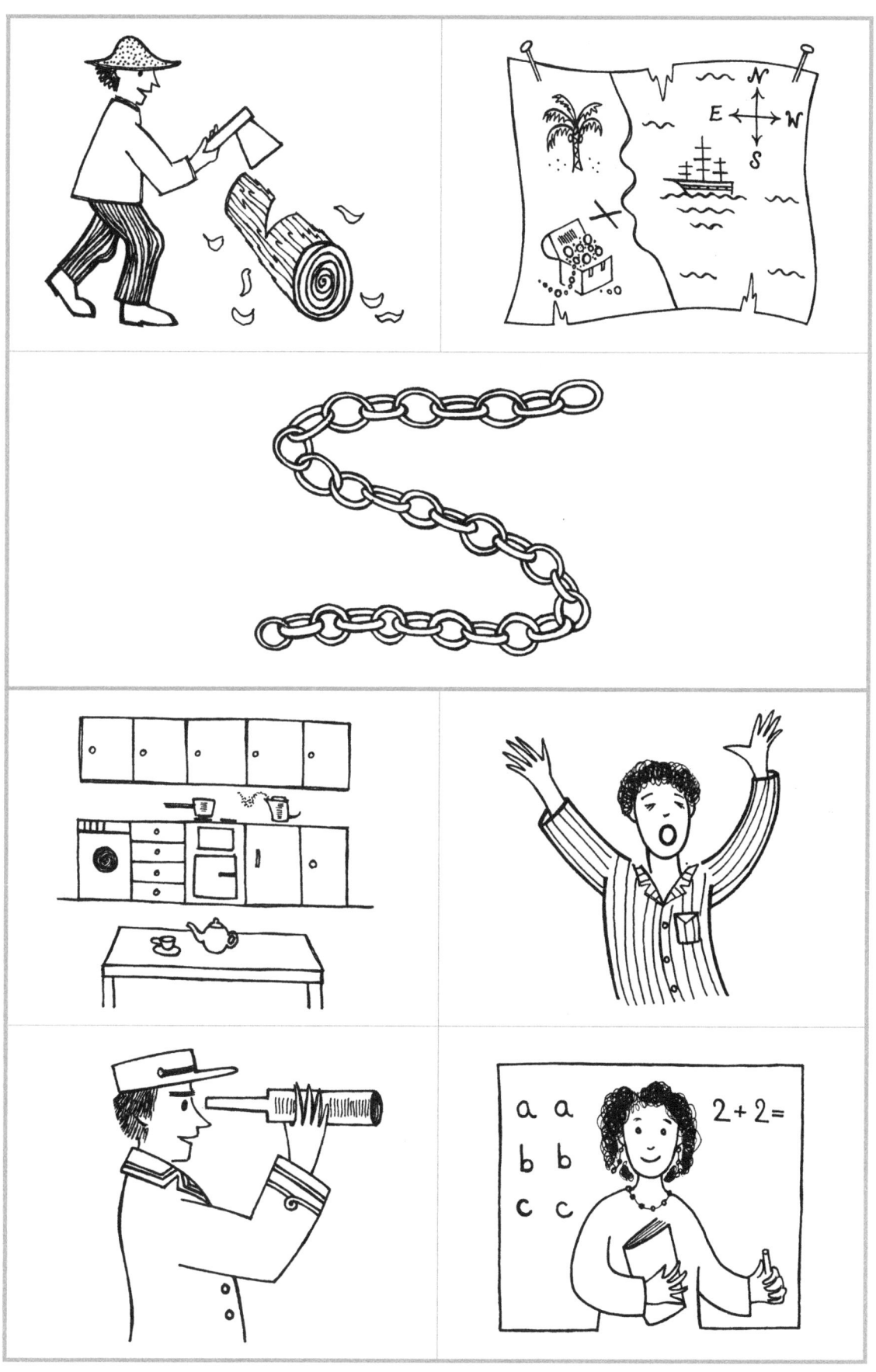

chop, chart, chain   kitchen, stretching, watching, teacher

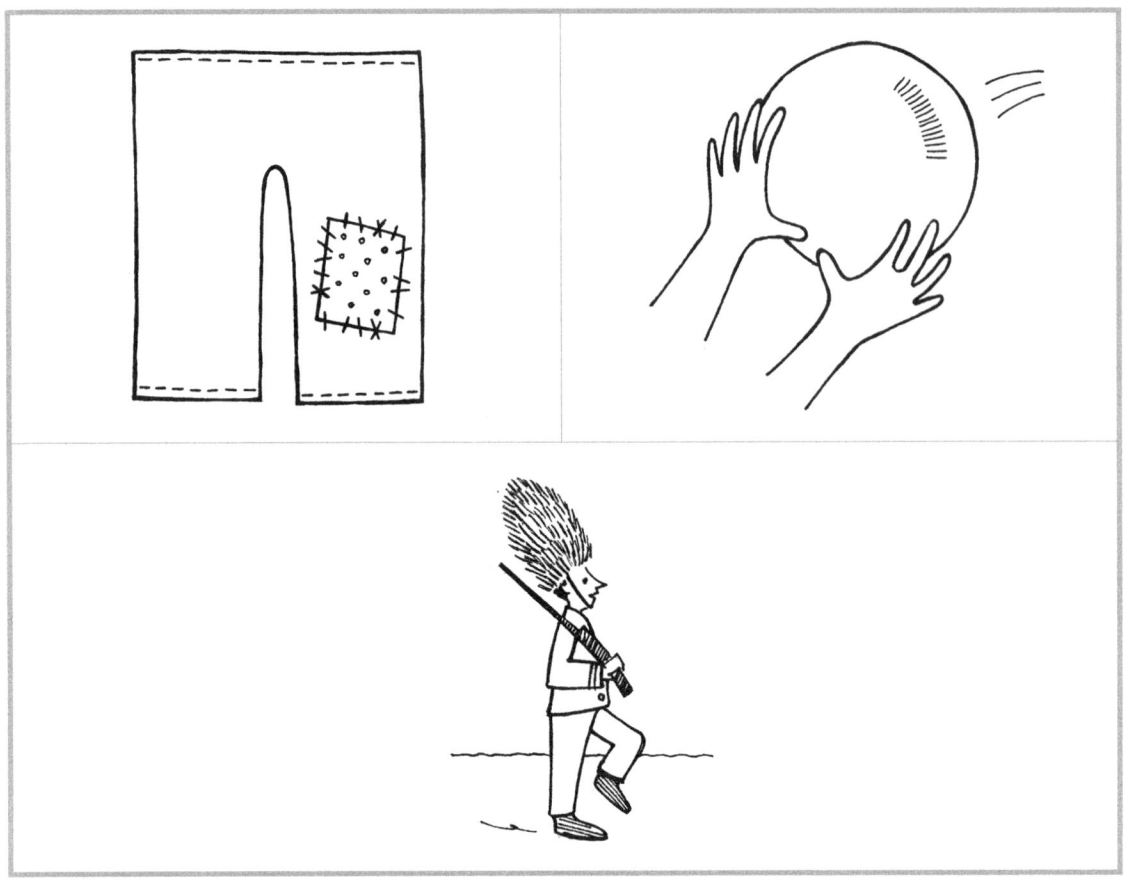

patch, catch, march

j

Word initial	Word medial	Word final
jam	urgent	**hedge**
jazz		lodge
jet	**magic**	**judge**
job	legend	
	logic	large
jar	reject	
jaw	project	wage
juice	budget	**page**
		rage
jail	region	huge
join		
joke	major	

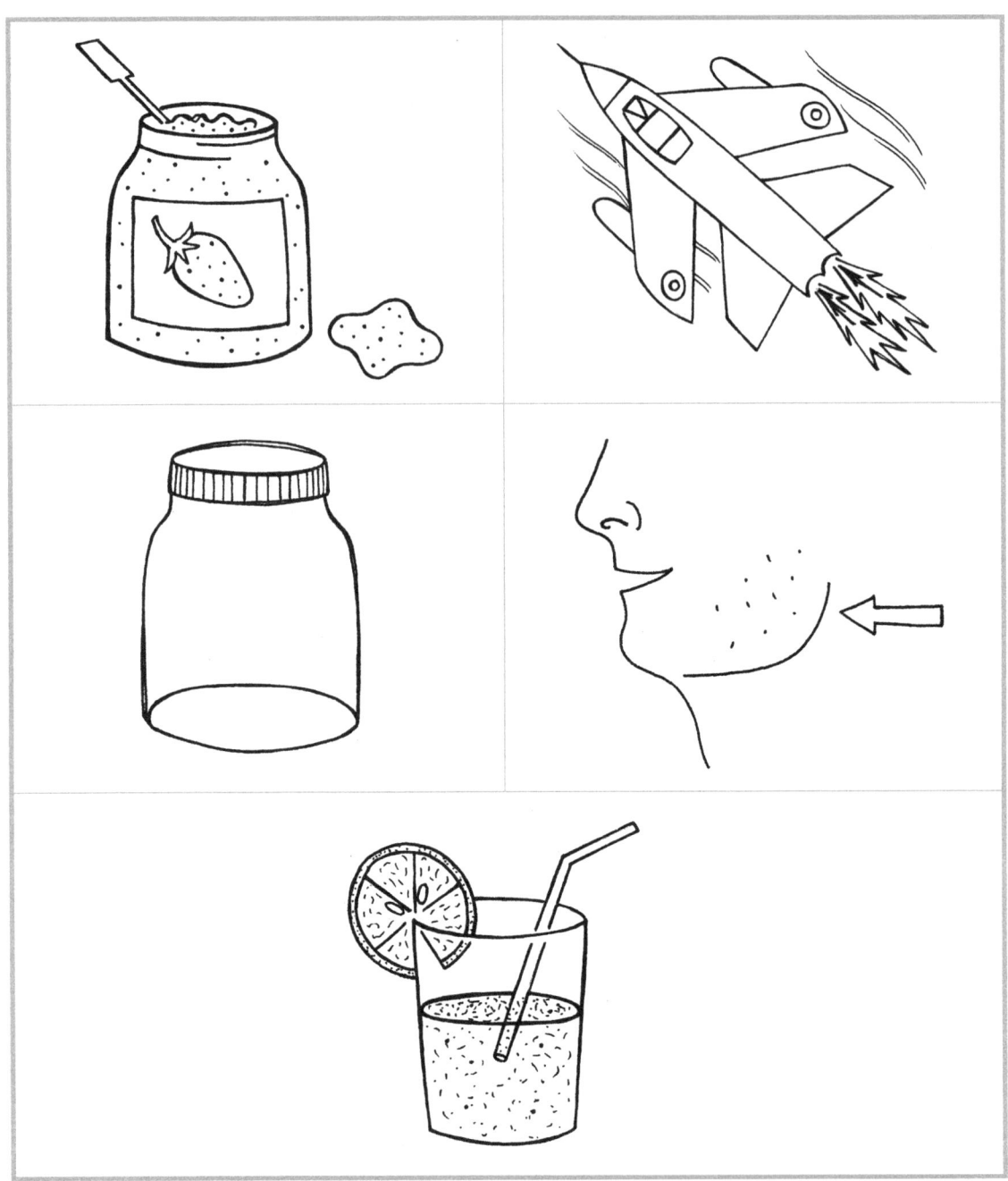

jam, jet, jar, jaw, juice

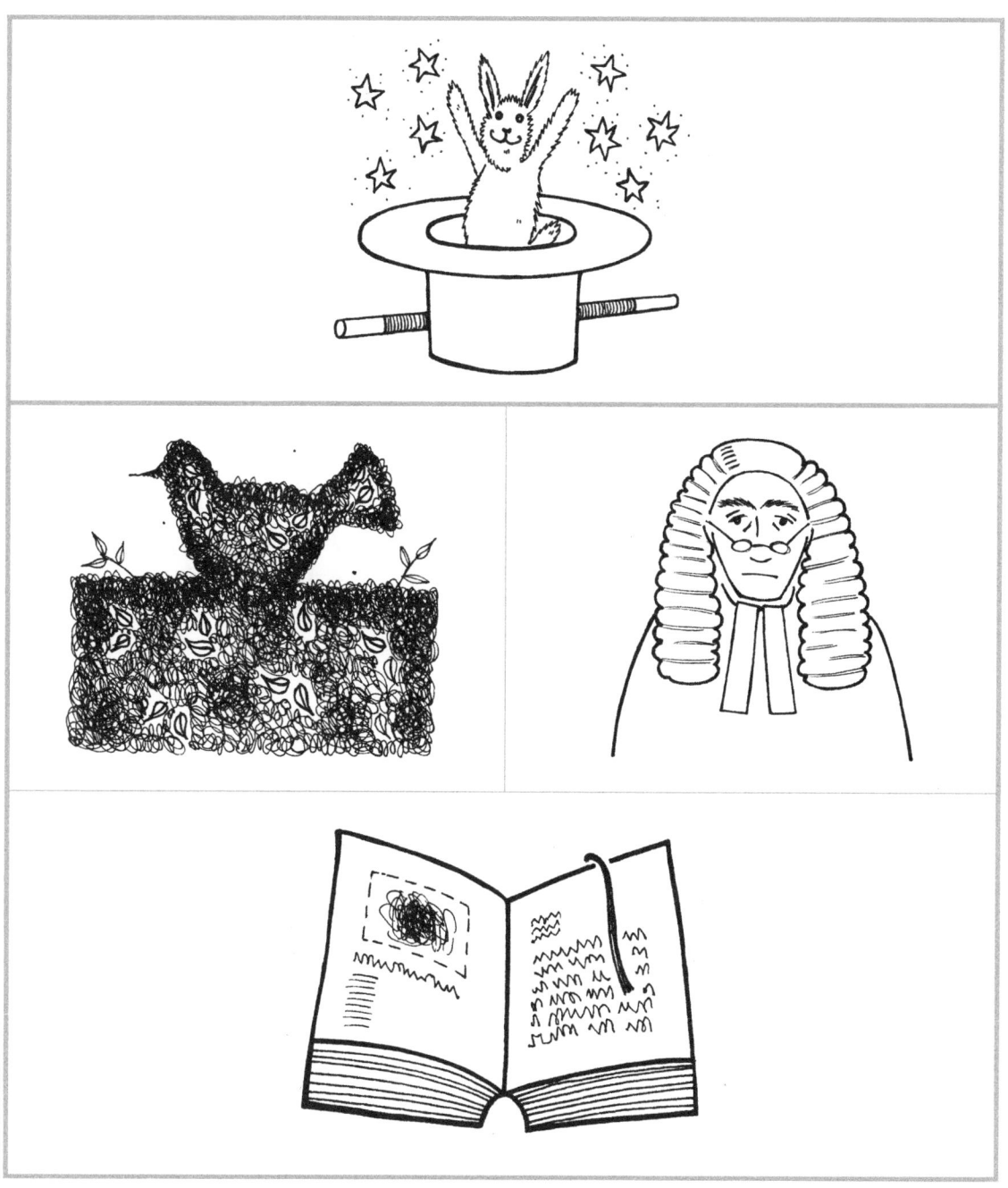

magic   hedge, judge   page

163

k

Word initial	Word medial	Word final
kiss	echo	thick
come		**neck**
cab	**chicken**	**back**
	jacket	dock
calm	**package**	**duck**
	lucky	**hook**
cake	**bucket**	
cave	decade	**park**
coal	pocket	
coat		folk
coin	**circle**	joke
	baker	
	broken	

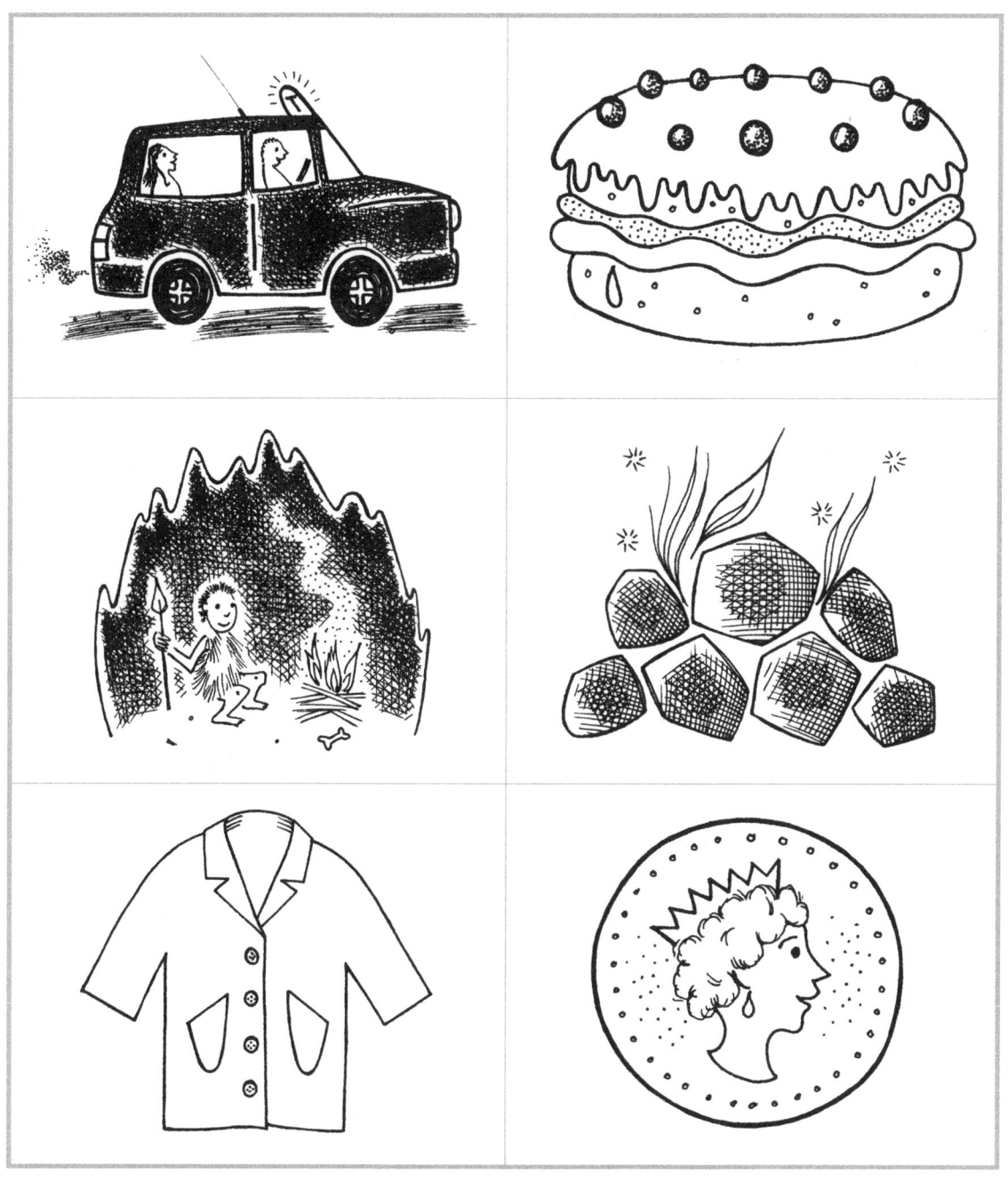

car, cake, cave, coal, coat, coin

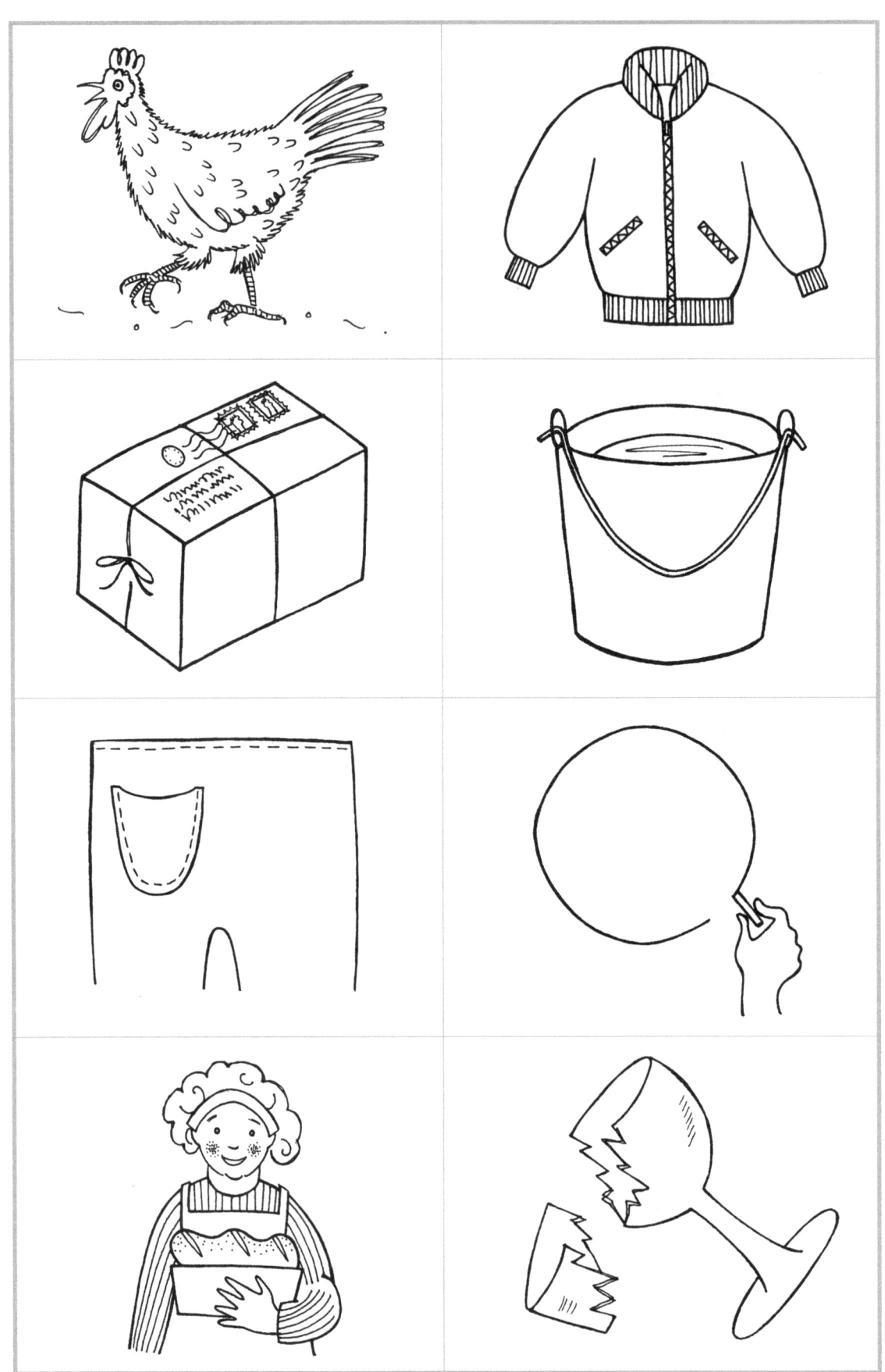

chicken, jacket, package, bucket, pocket, circle, baker, broken

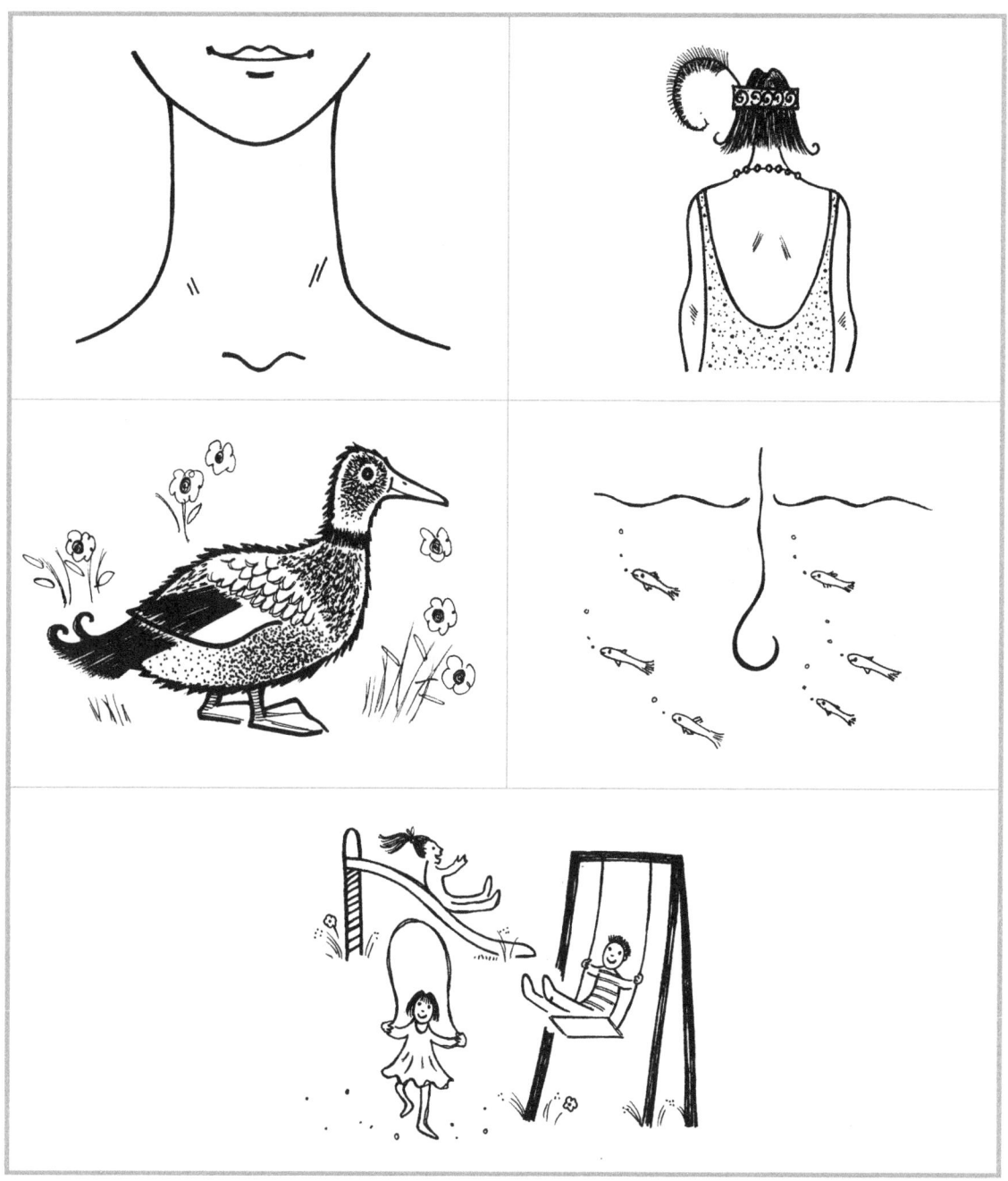

neck, back, duck, hook, park

g

Word initial	Word medial	Word final
get	**eagle**	**pig**
gas	**organ**	big
gap		**mug**
god	begin	fog
good	bigger	
give	figure	vague
	forgive	
girl		
guard	legal	
	target	
gaze		
gate		

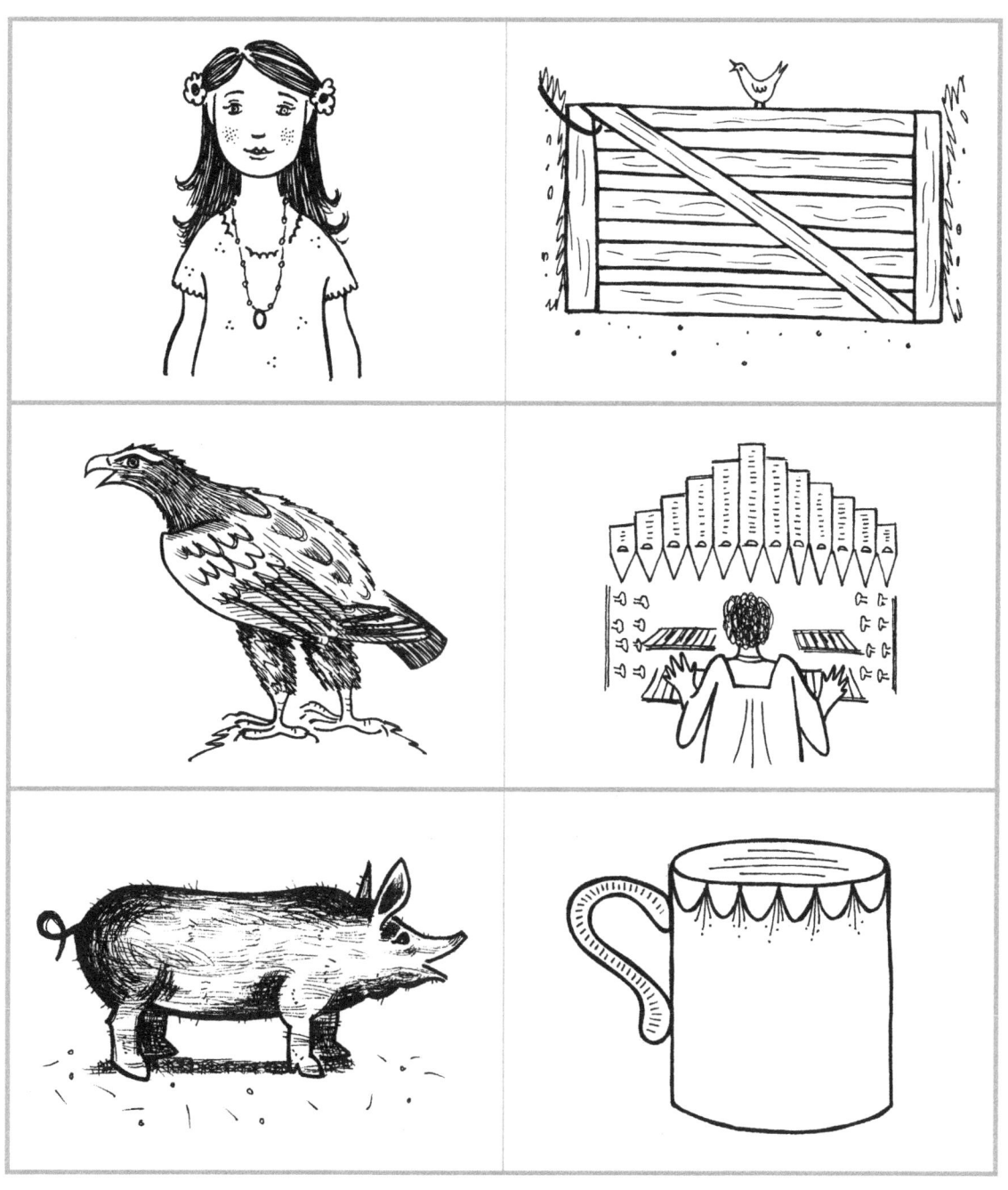

girl, gate   eagle, organ   pig, mug

l	

Word initial	Word medial	Word final
leg	alarm	hill
lip		
lad	villa	fool
	filling	pool
lead	belong	**ball**
learn	believe	
lawn	delay	**coal**
lord	valid	**bowl**
loop	colour	**meal**
	collar	seal
loan	follow	pale
life		**tail**
lace	calling	
	falling	
	ceiling	
	foolish	

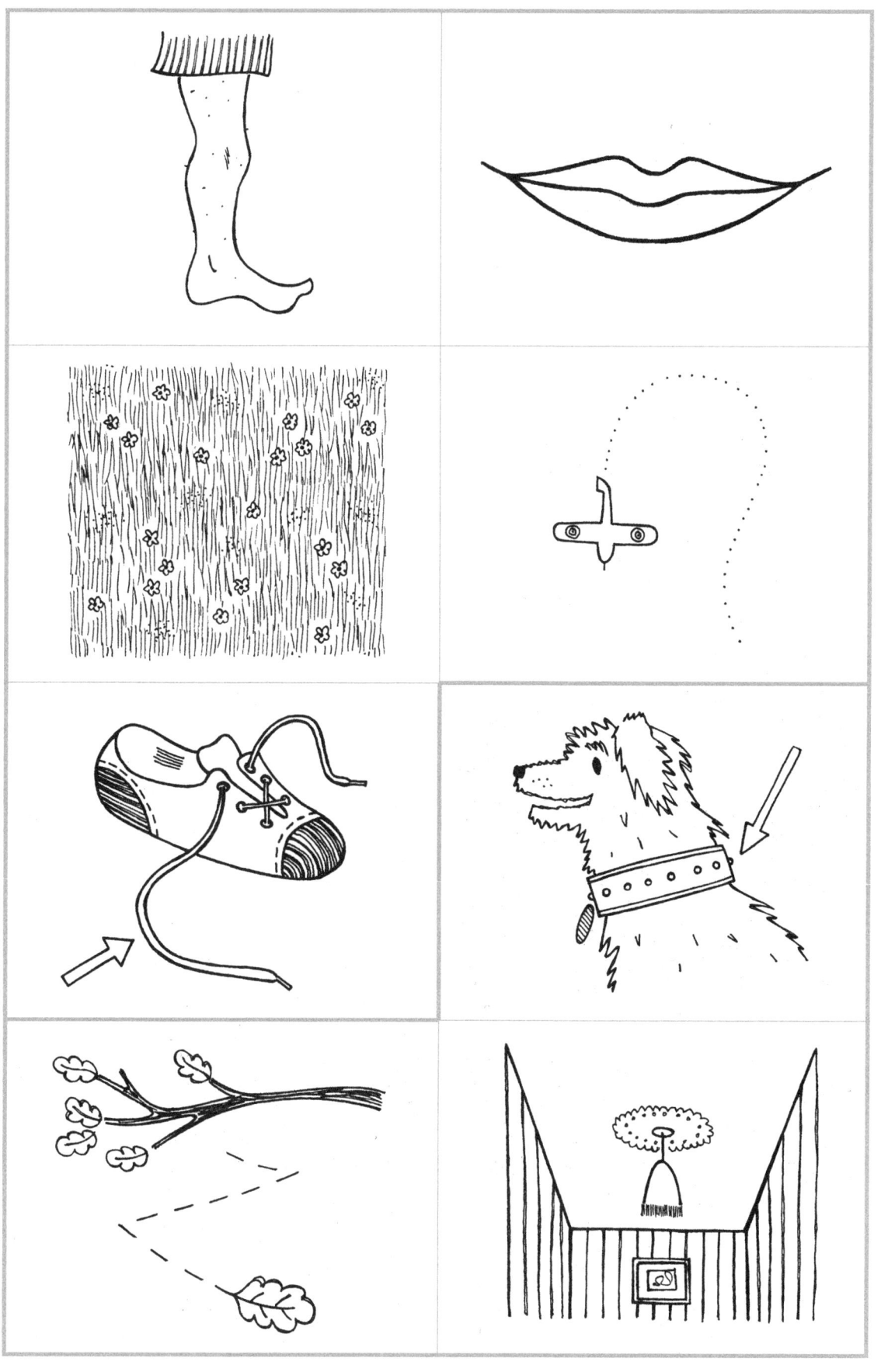

leg, lip, lawn, loop, lace   collar, falling, ceiling

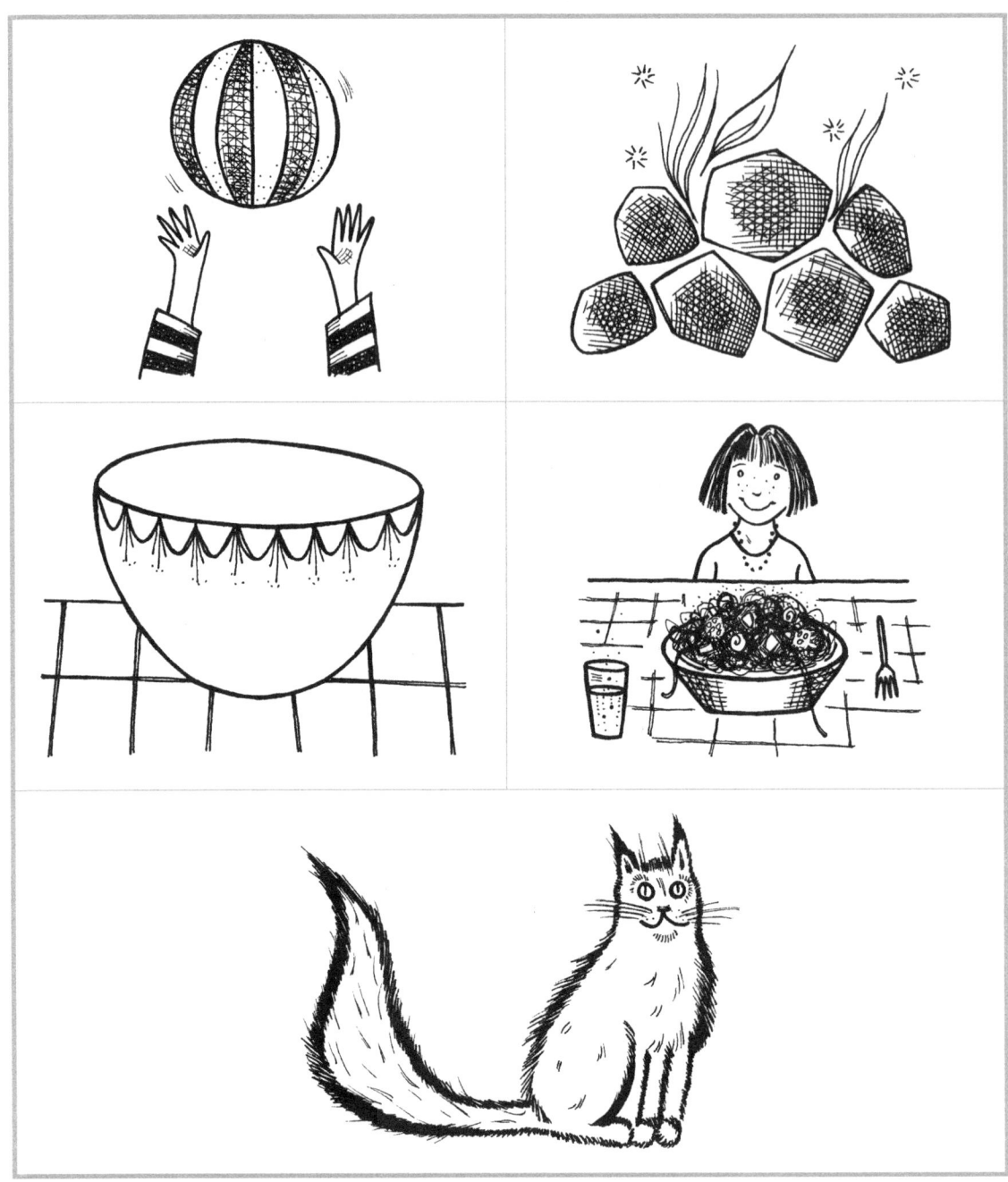

ball, coal, bowl, meal, tail

r

Word initial	Word medial	Word final
rid	borrow	
rat	**forest**	
rock	moral	
	career	
reach	parade	
room	**carriage**	
	current	
rage		
rain	hero	
right	virus	
rose		

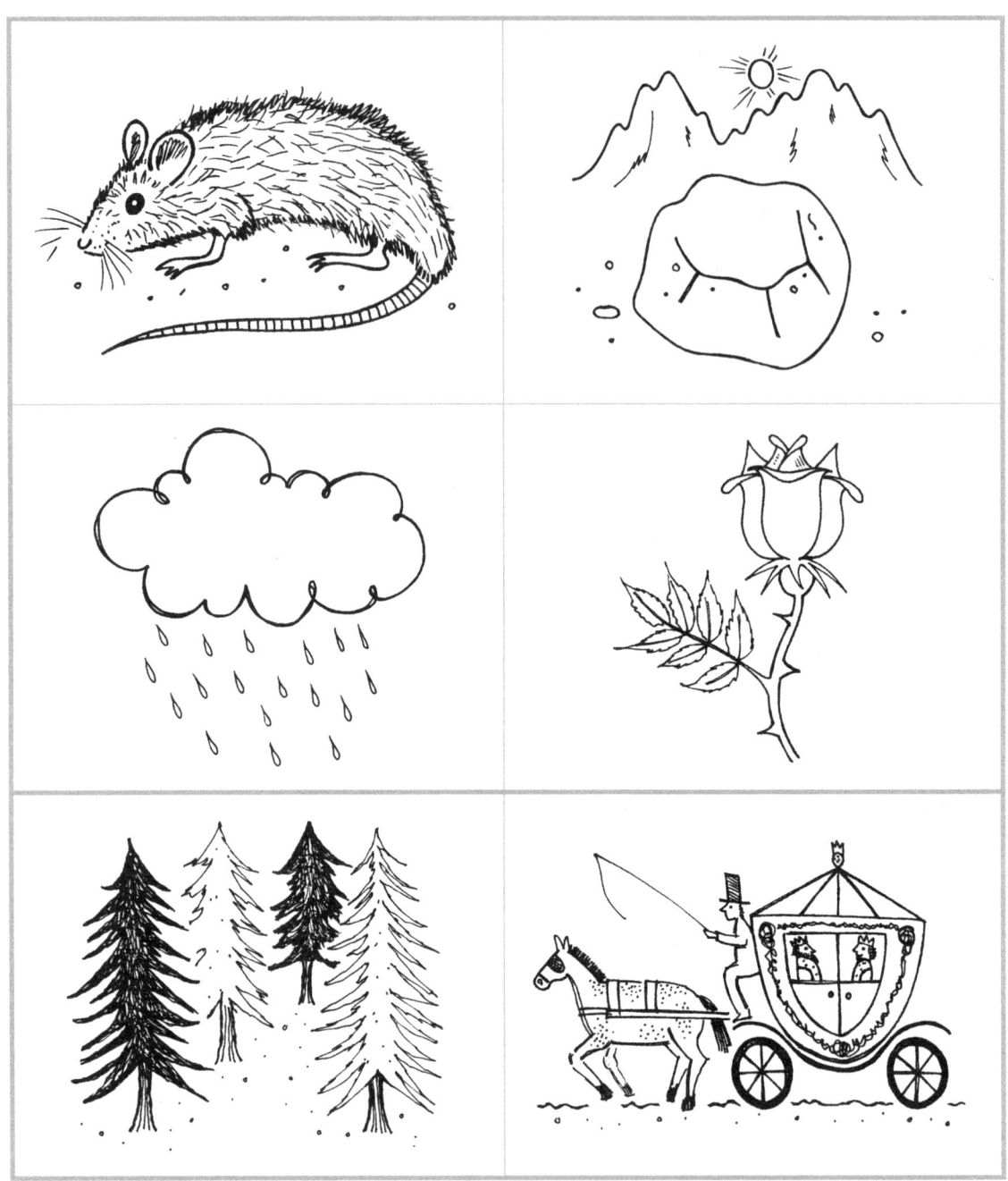

rat, rock, rain, rose   forest, carriage

Word initial	Word medial	Word final
wet	reward	
win		
wish	chewing	
what		
	power	
wheat	**shower**	
work	**flower**	
walk	**tower**	
	knowing	
wage		
wide		

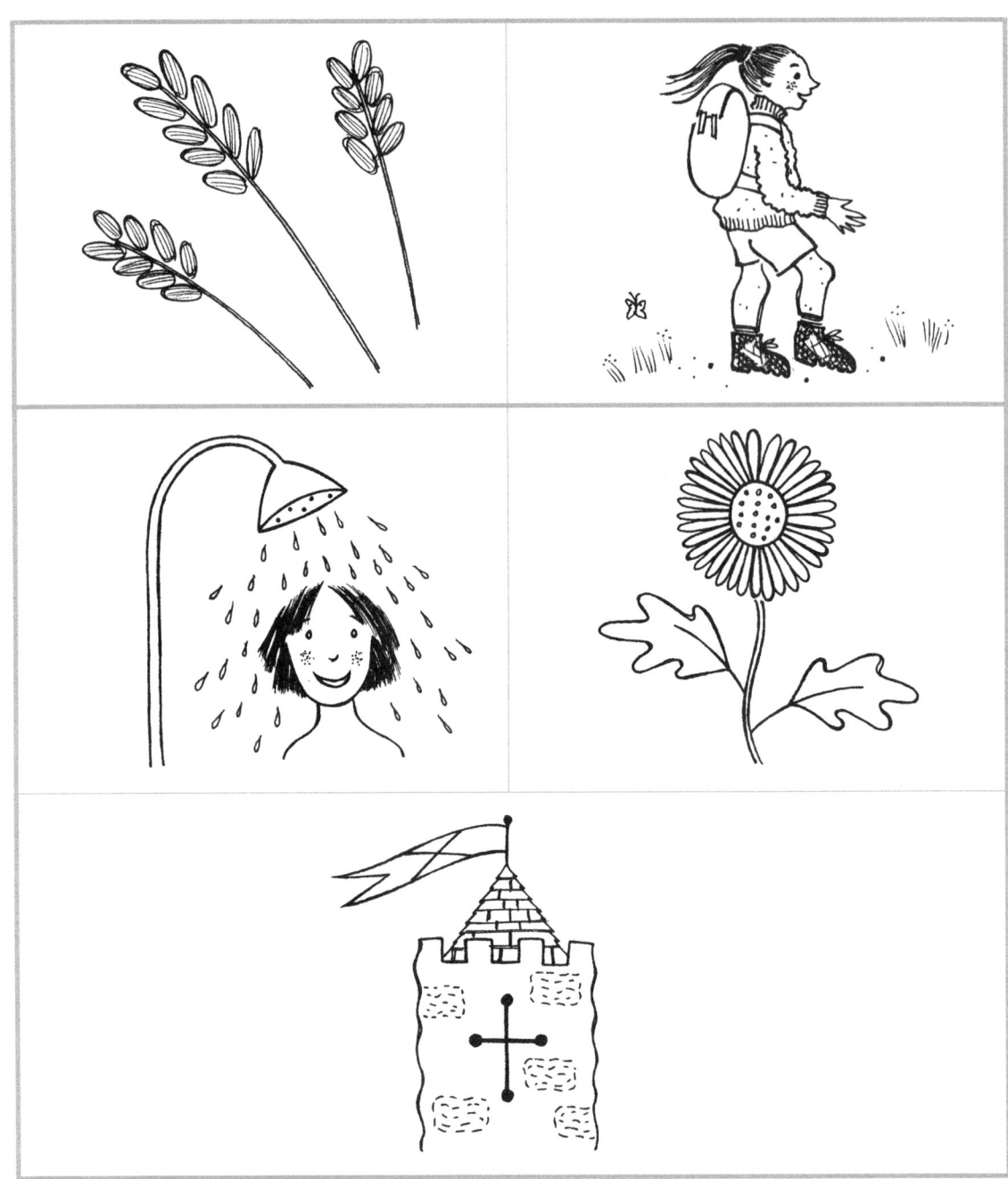

wheat, walk   shower, flower, tower

y

Word initial	Word medial	Word final
yes		
yet		
young		
yacht		
yard		
youth		

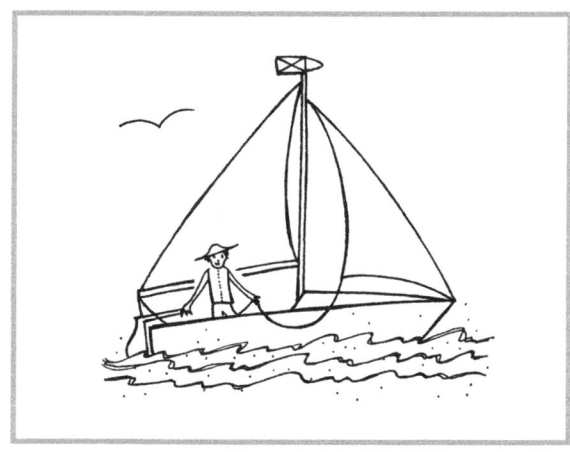

yacht

h

Word initial	Word medial	Word final
hip	behave	
head	behind	
hot		
hook		
heat		
horn		
hurt		
heart		
height		
hope		

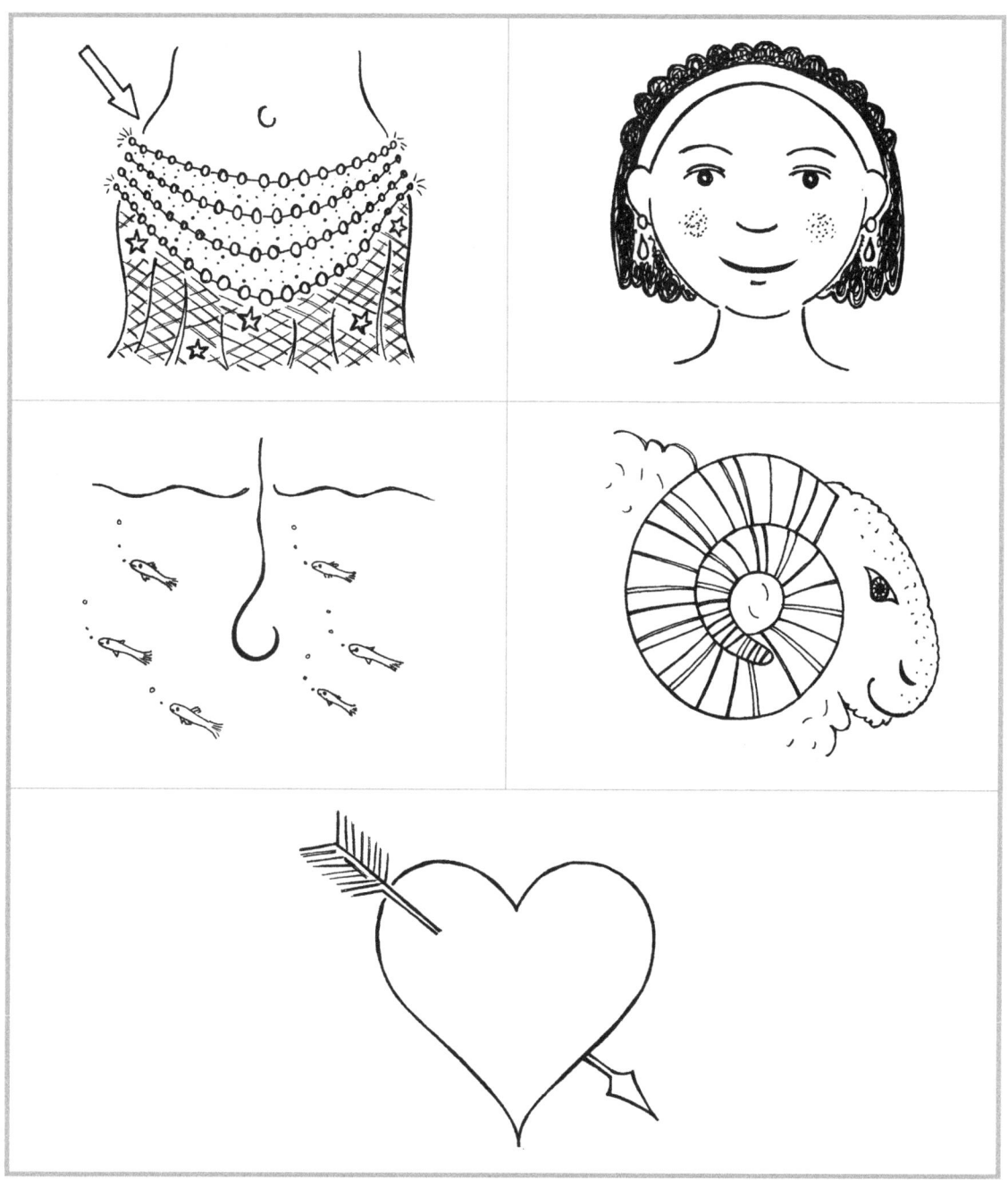

hip, head, hook, horn, heart

Word initial	Word medial	Word final
	finger	king
	singing	wing
	bringing	gang
		long
		wrong
		young
		tongue
		reading

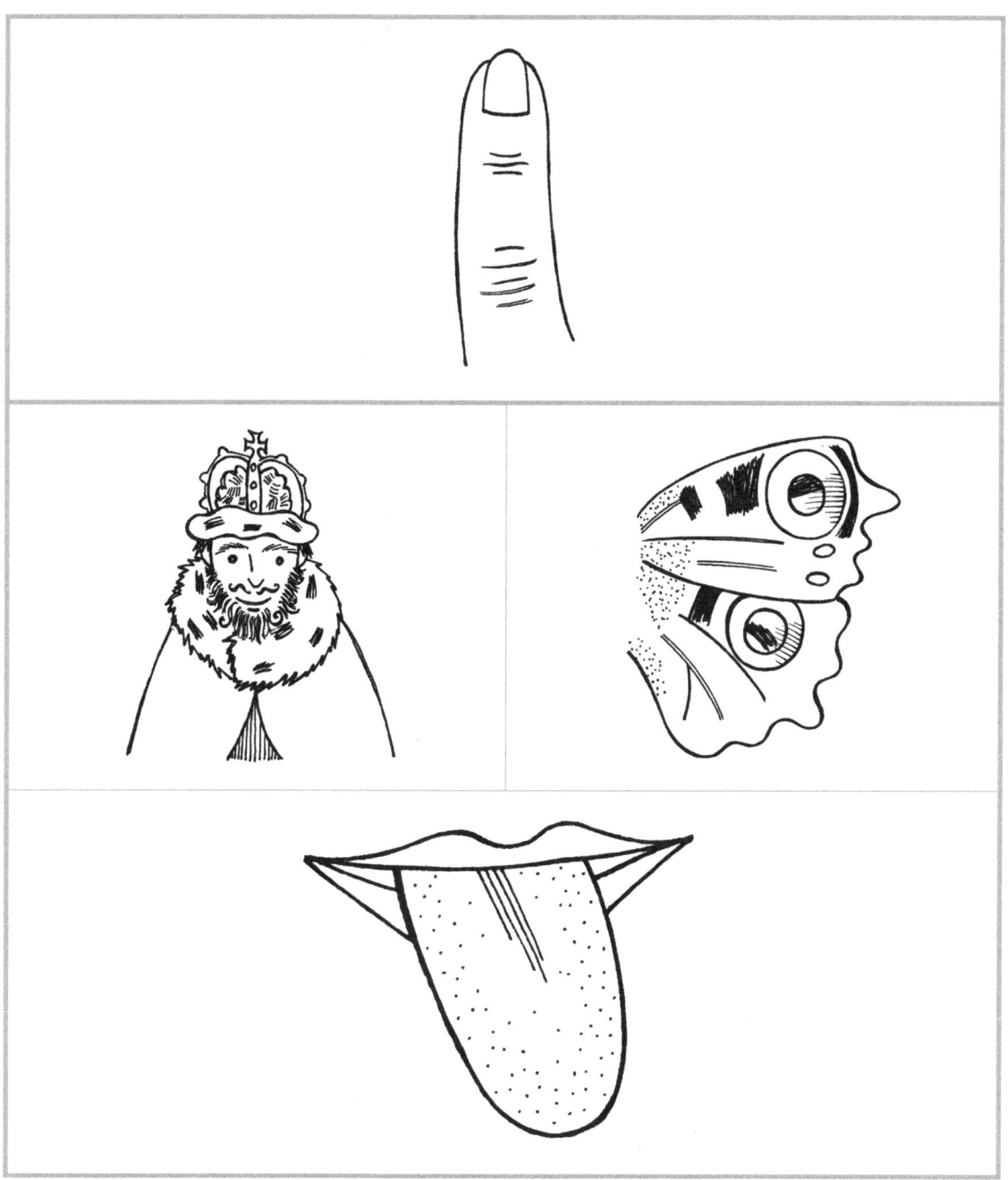

finger   king, wing   tongue

pl	pr
pleasure	press
plan	print
plastic	
plant	**priest**
plot	proof
please	pray
	praise
place	prayer
plate	price
plain	**prize**
	proud

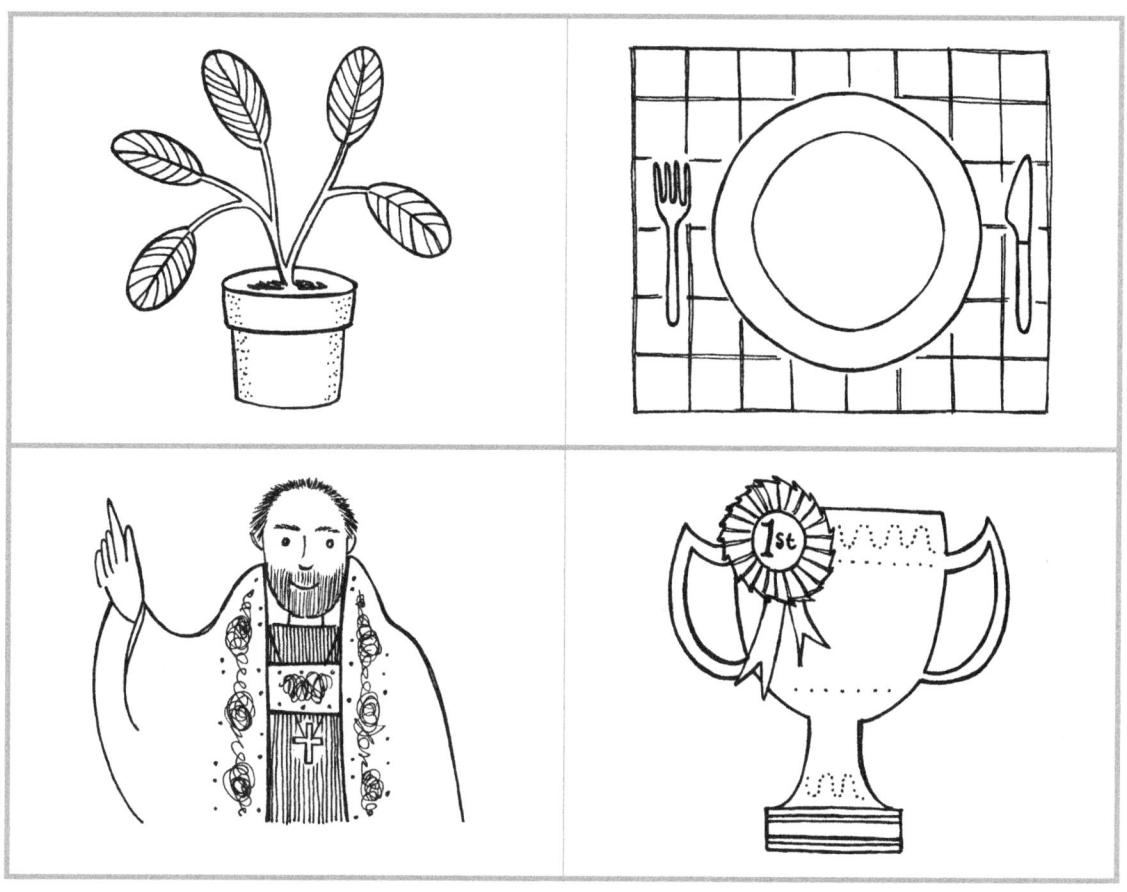

plant, plate   priest, prize

bl	br
black	**bread**
blank	breath
block	**bridge**
blood	**branch**
	brand
blade	brass
blame	**brush**
blind	
blow	breeze
bloke	
	break
	brave
	brain
	bride

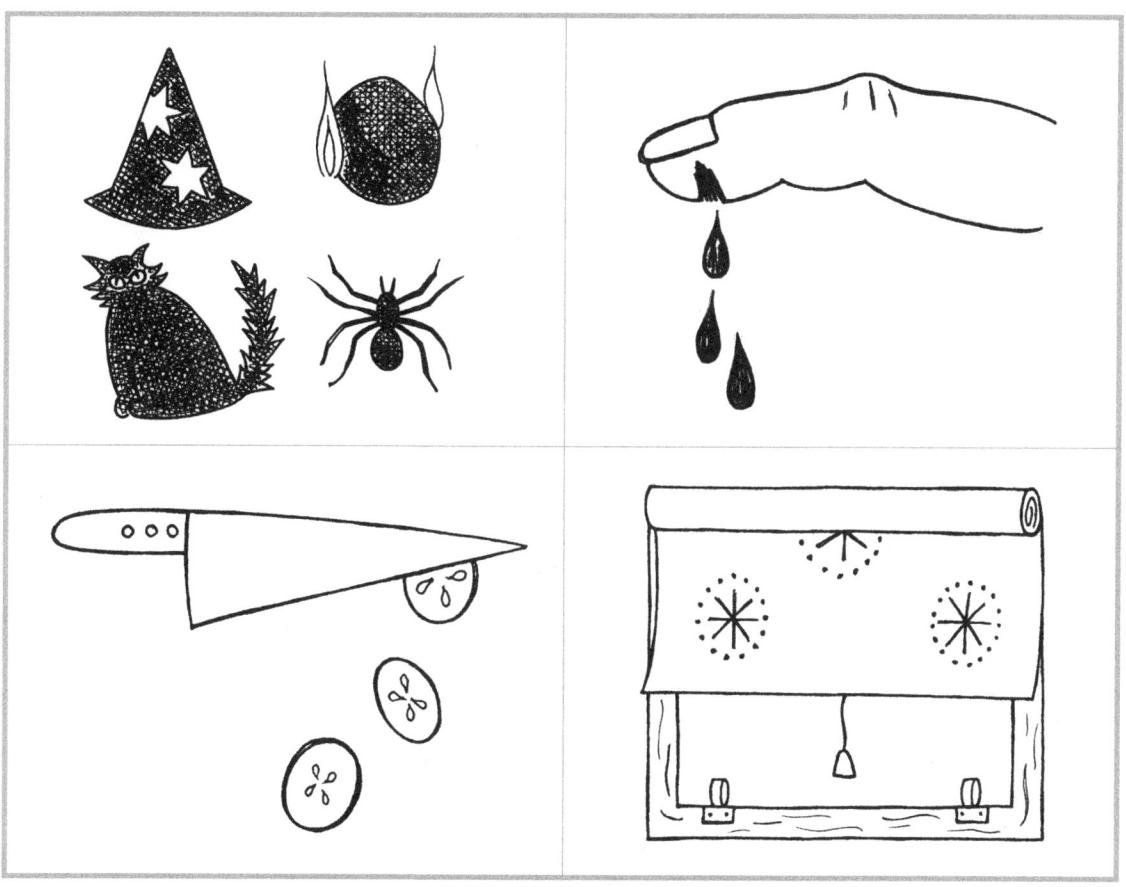

black, blood, blade, blind

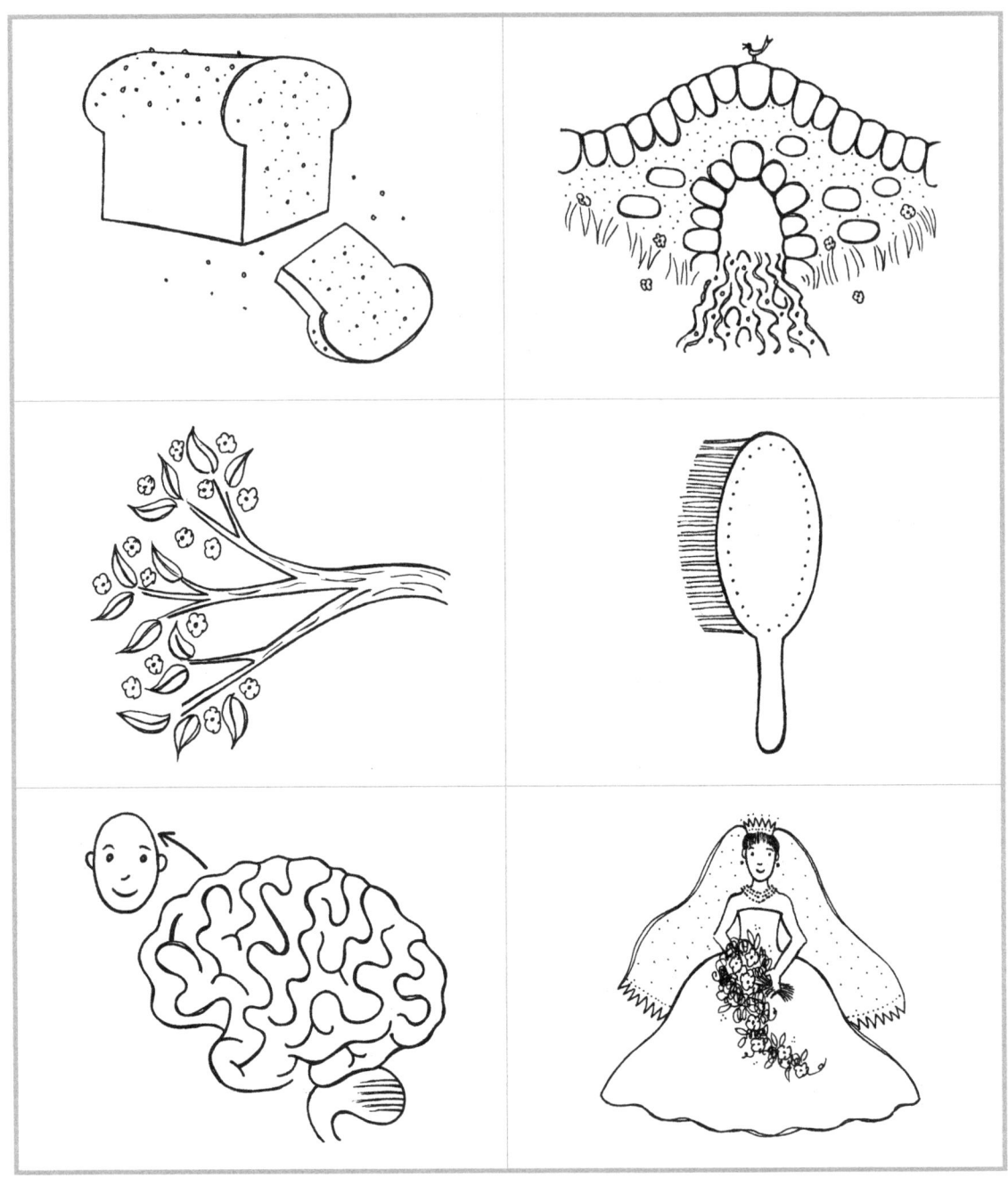

bread, bridge, branch, brush, brain, bride

fl	fr
flesh	fresh
flat	friend
flood	**fringe**
	front
fleet	France
floor	
	fruit
flame	frequent
fly	
flight	**frame**
flour	Friday
flow	

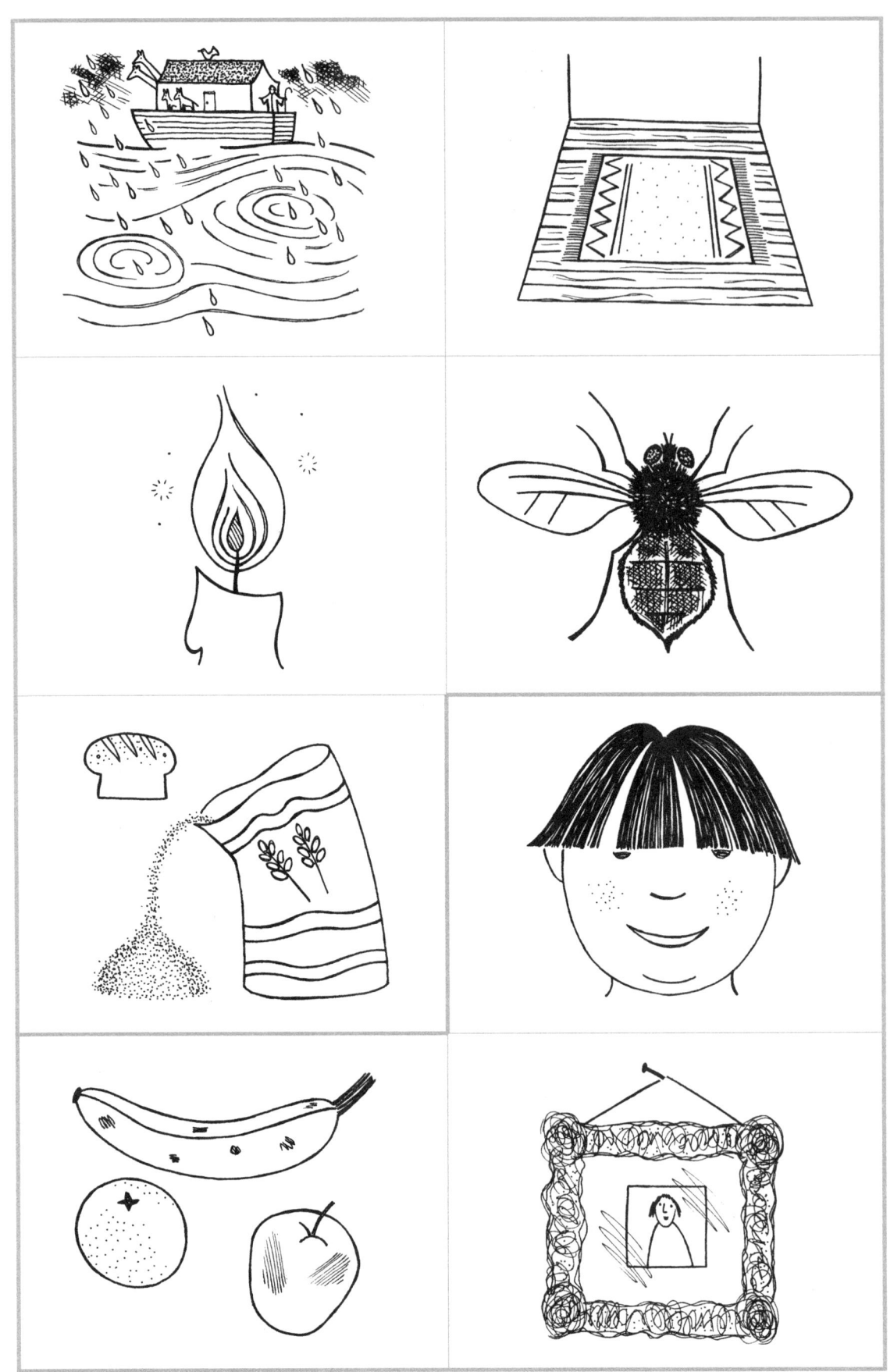

flood, floor, flame, fly, flour   fringe, fruit, frame

thr

threat
thrust
through
throw
throne
throat

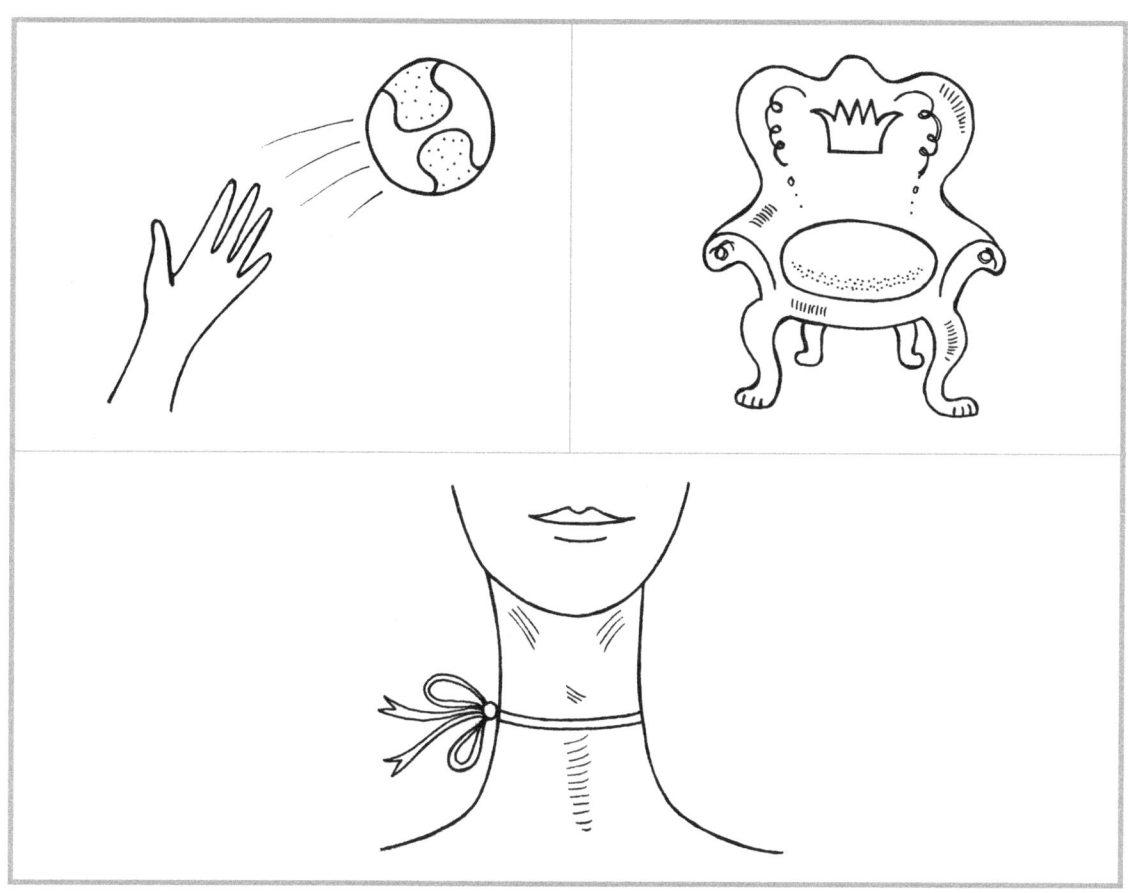

throw, throne, throat

tr

trap
track
truck
trick
tree
treat
tray
trace
train
trial
trousers

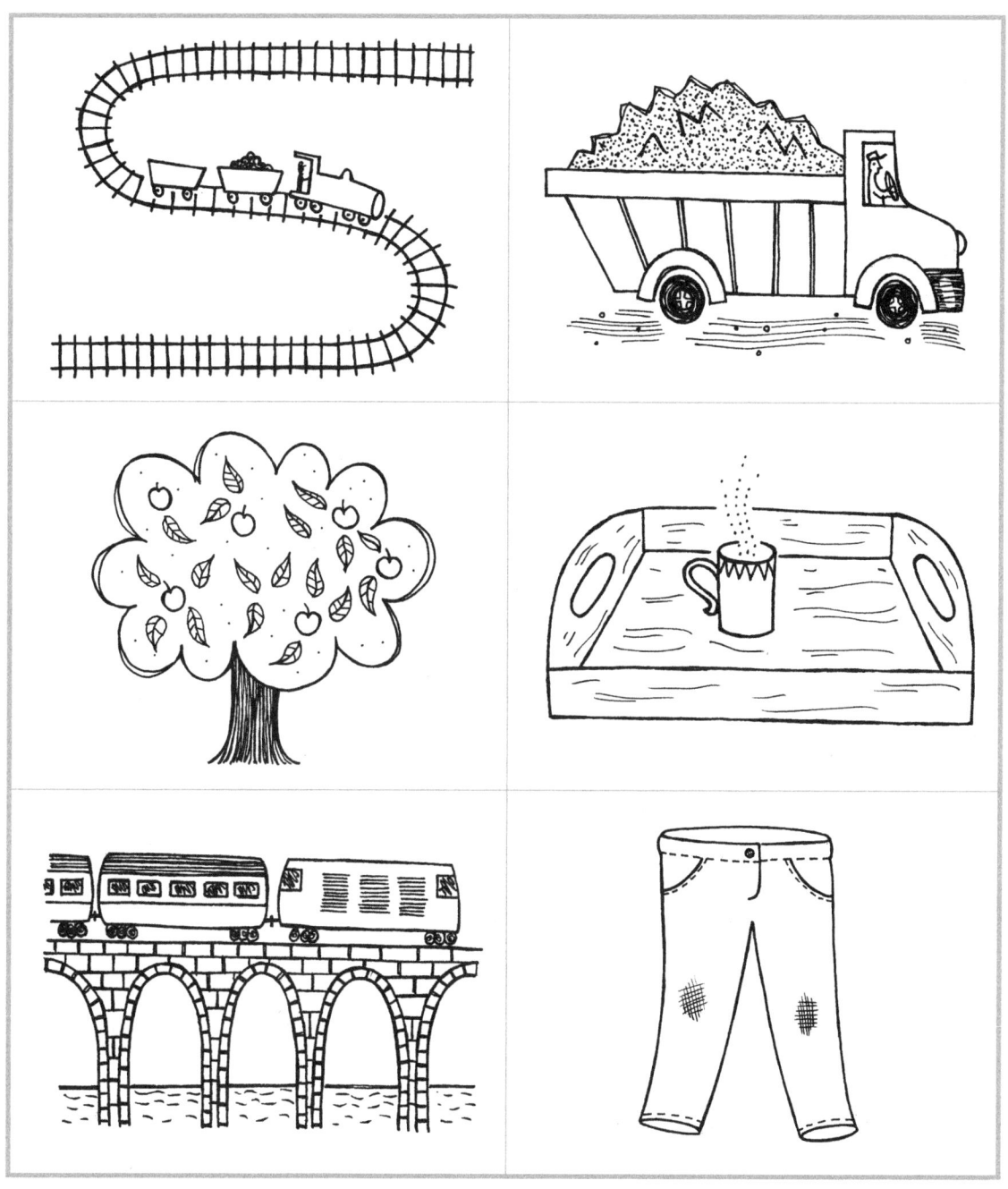

track, truck, tree, tray, train, trousers

dress
drop
drug
drunk
draft
drink
drawer
dream
drive

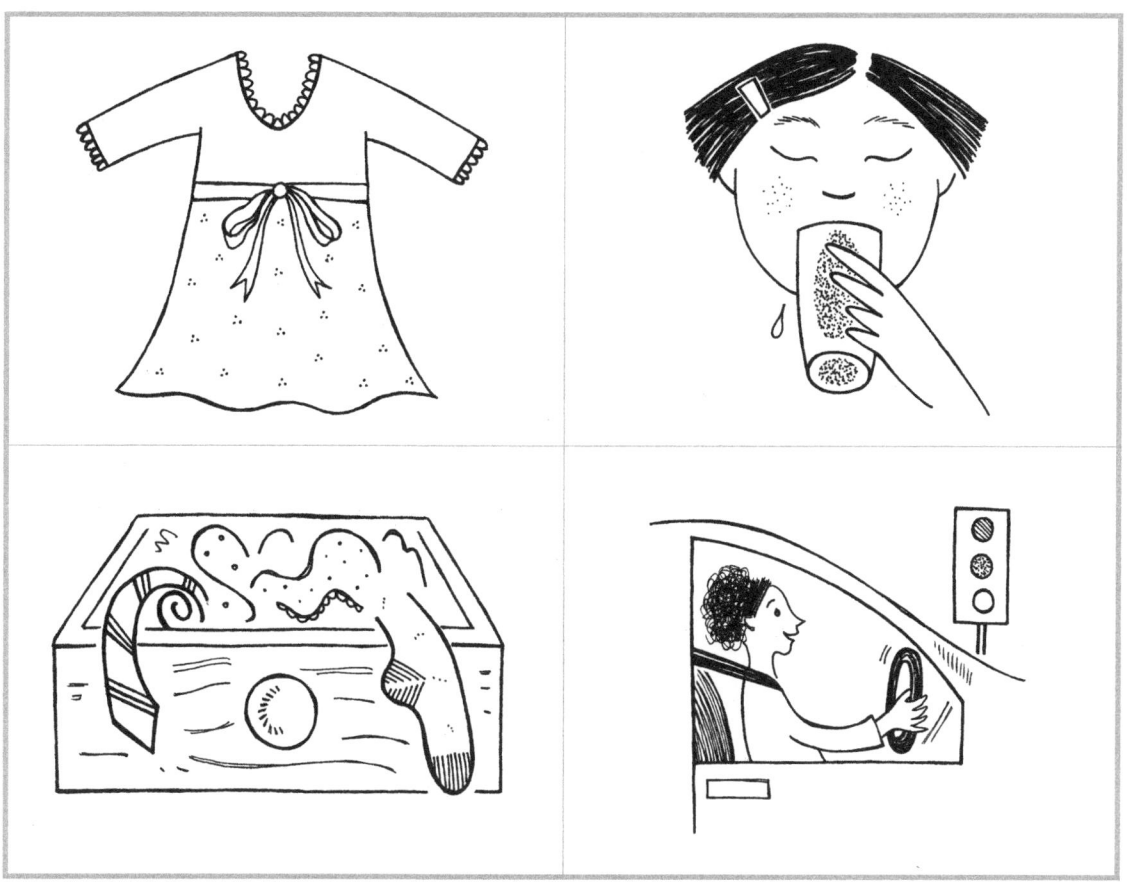

dress, drink, drawer, drive

kl	kr	kw
clever	**crash**	quick
clock	credit	**quid**
cliff	**cross**	
class	**cricket**	quite
	crystal	quiet
clean		quote
	cream	
claim		
climb	**cry**	
clothes	cruel	
close	**crowd**	

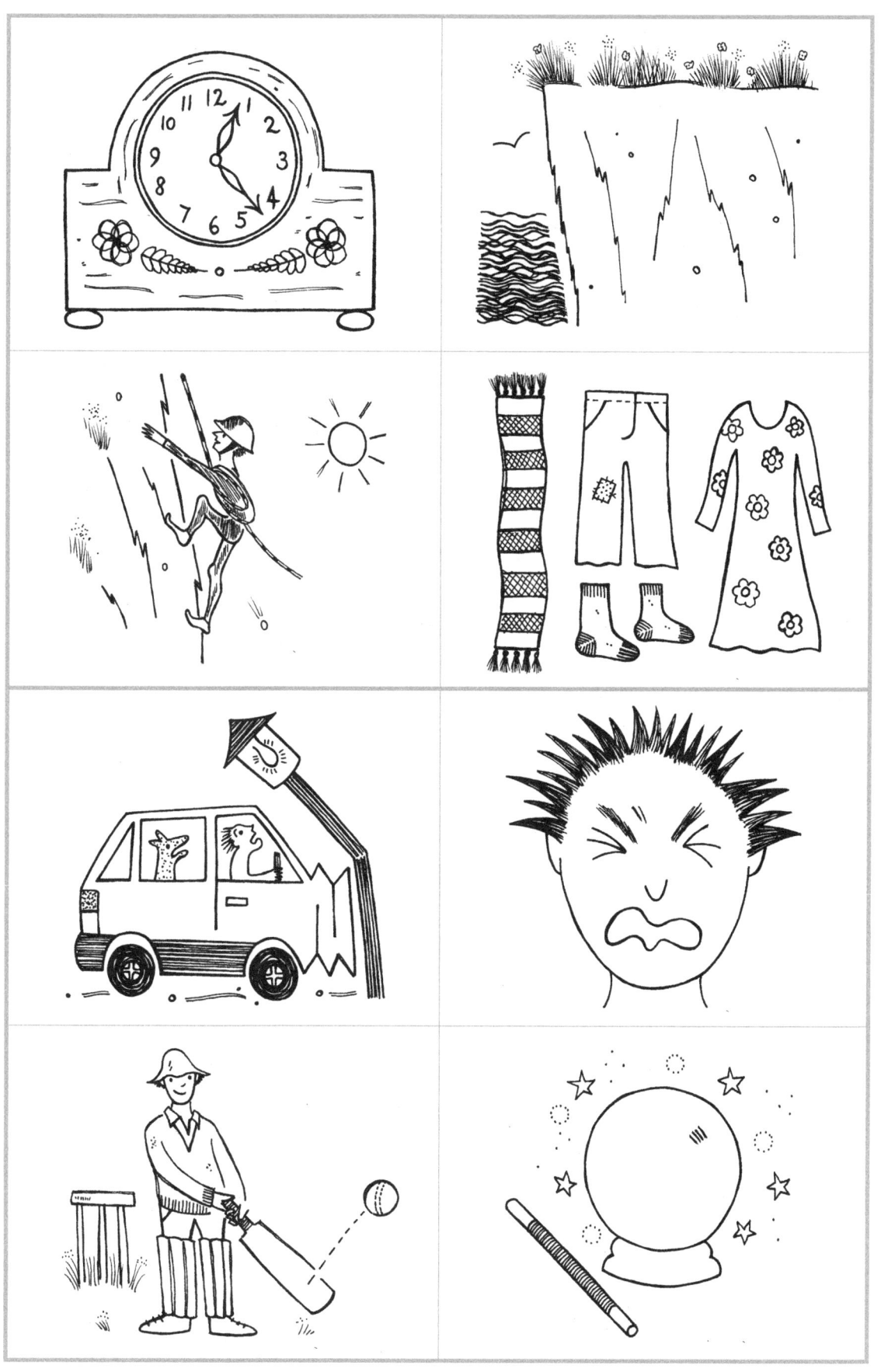

clock, cliff, climb, clothes   crash, cross, cricket, crystal

Clusters /kr/ and /kw/

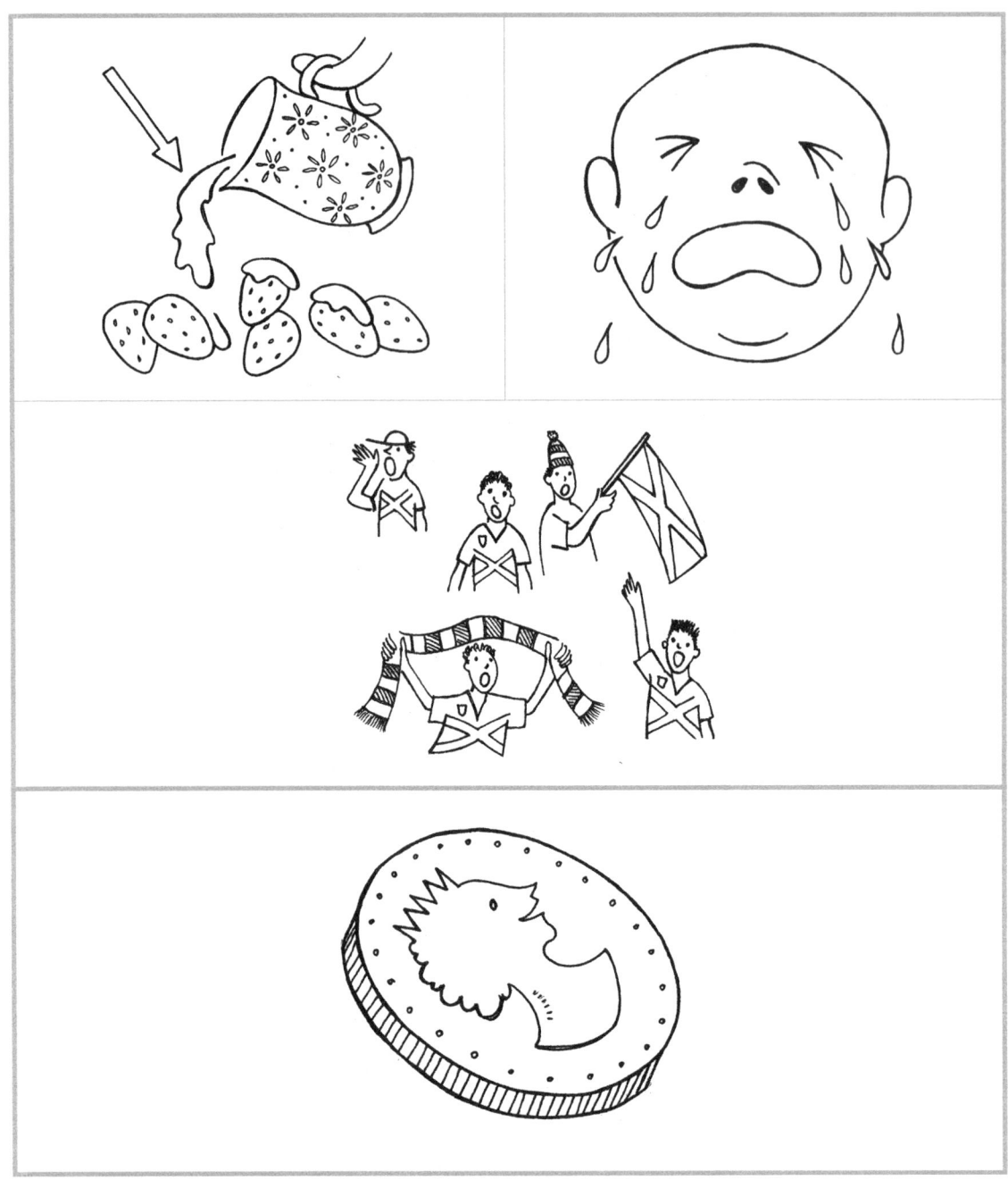

cream, cry, crowd   quid

gl	gr
glass	**grid**
glad	grin
glance	**graph**
gloves	grand
glory	**green**
	group
global	
	grey
	grace
	great
	grow
	ground

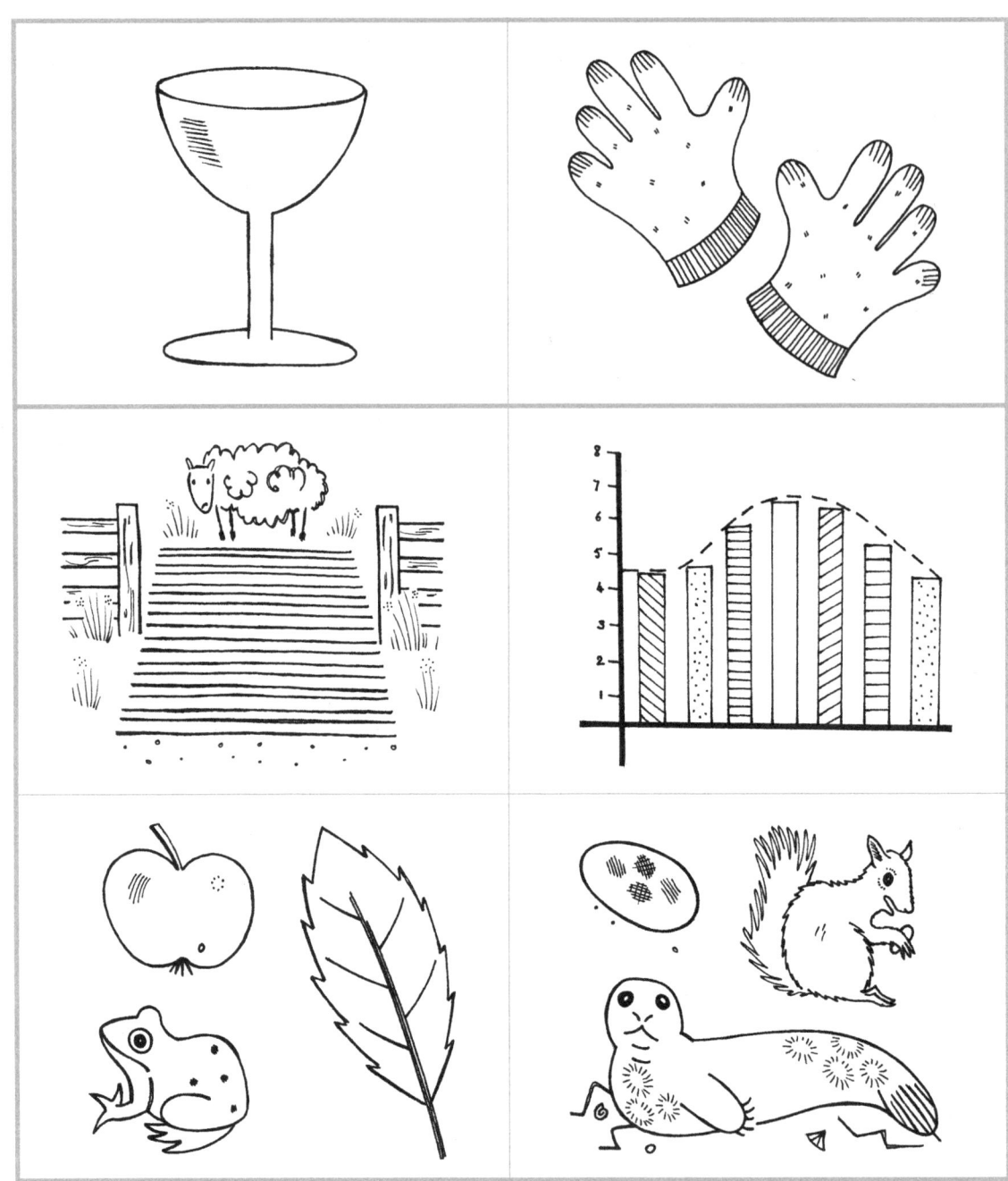

glass, gloves   grid, graph, green, grey

sl	sm	sn
slim	smell	sniff
slip		snap
	smart	snatch
sleep	**small**	
sleeve	smooth	**snake**
		snow
slide		
slow		

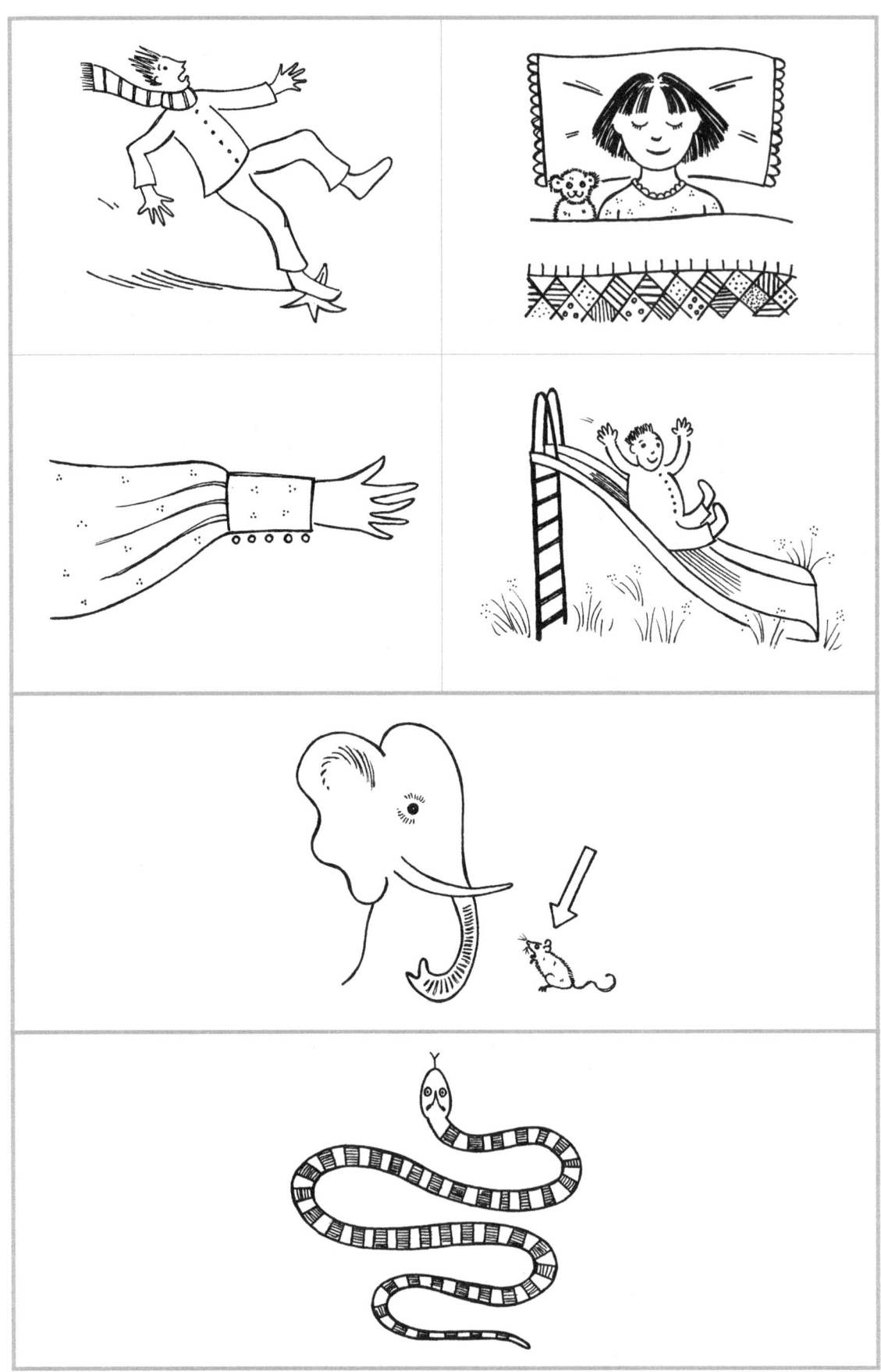

slip, sleep, sleeve, slide   small   snake

sp	st	sk
spell	staff	skin
spot	**stamp**	skill
spirit	stand	**skull**
	stick	skirt
speak	study	
speed		
sport	**star**	
	start	
Spain	**storm**	
space		
spine	steel	
spare	**stable**	
	stage	
	stairs	
	stone	

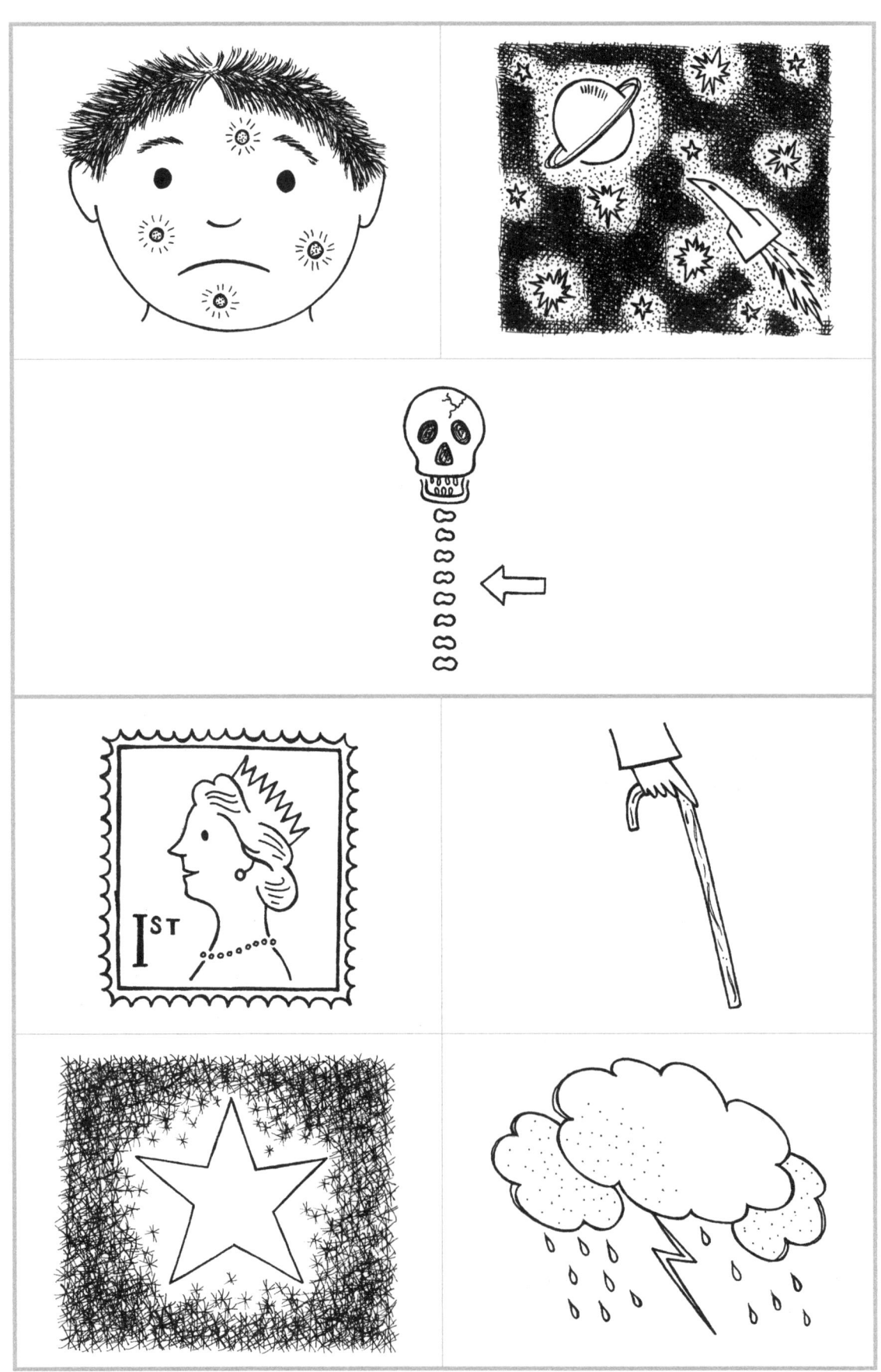

spots, space, spine   stamp, stick, star, storm

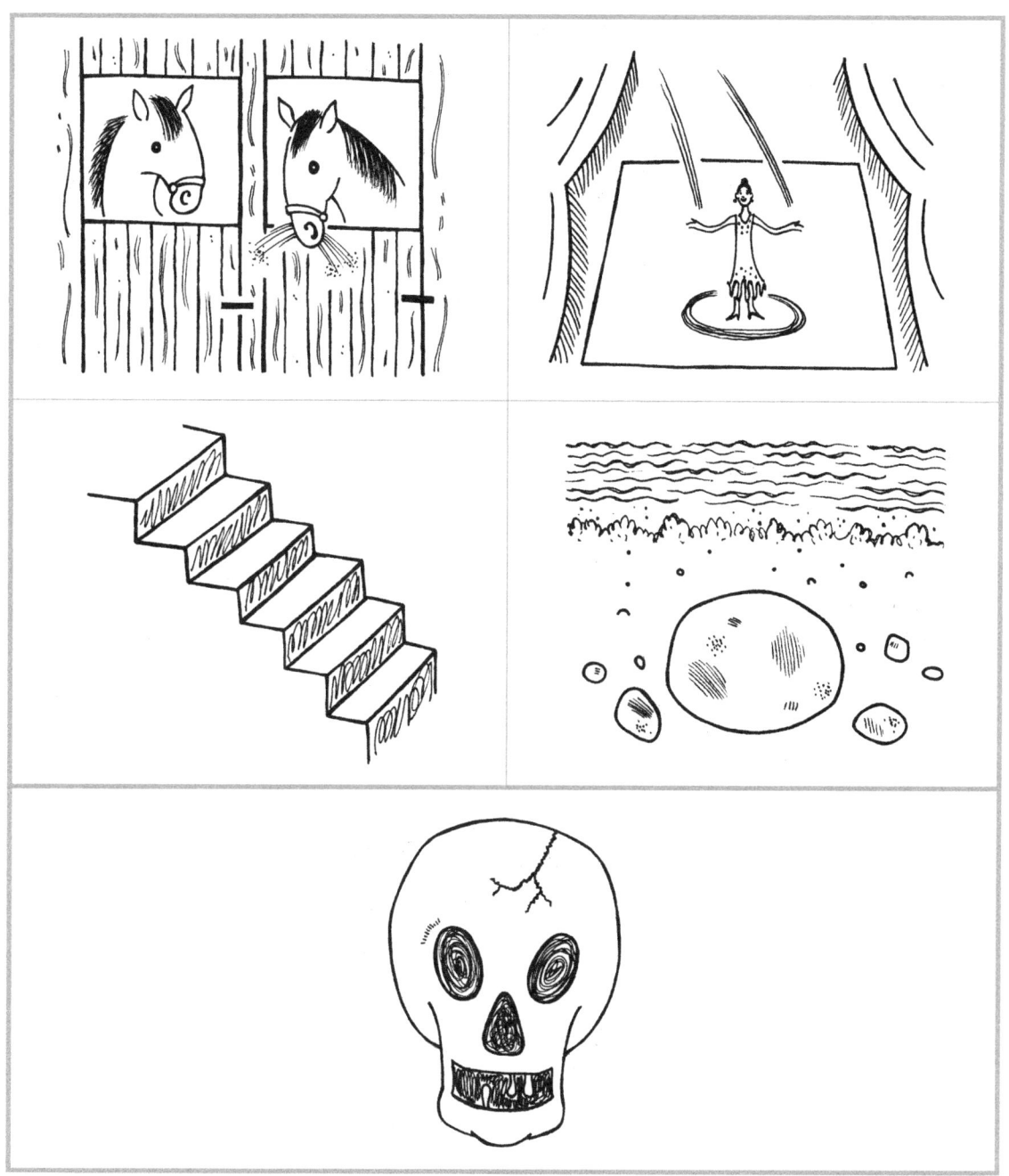

stable, stage, stairs, stone   skull

| switch |
| **swing** |
| Swiss |
| swiftly |
| **swim** |
| sweet |
| Sweden |

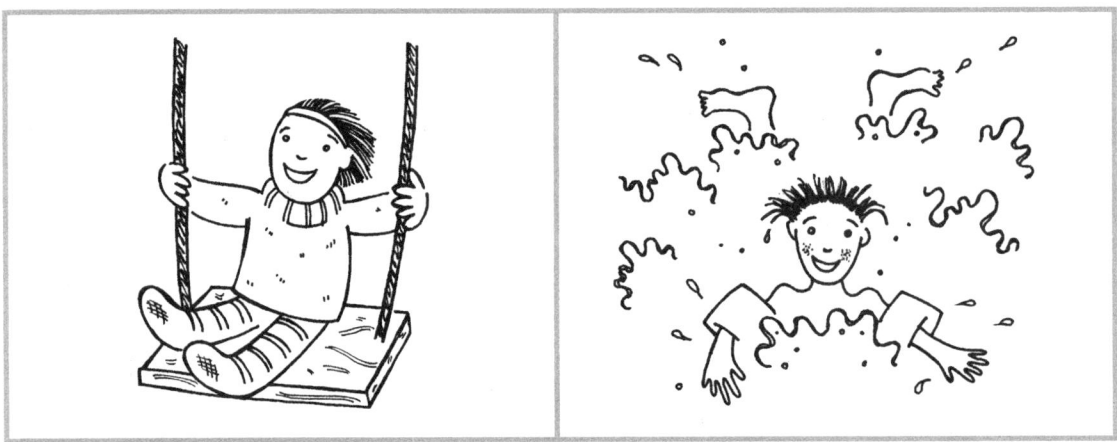

swing, swim

LEVEL 6 Multisyllabic words

2 syllable words
3 or more syllable words

LEVEL 6 presents all English consonants in word initial position of multisyllabic words. Pictures of imageable words are presented. Words lists and pictures can be photocopied for speech practice.

2 syllable words

package
pushing
people
pardon
portion
purchase
power
pupil
parade

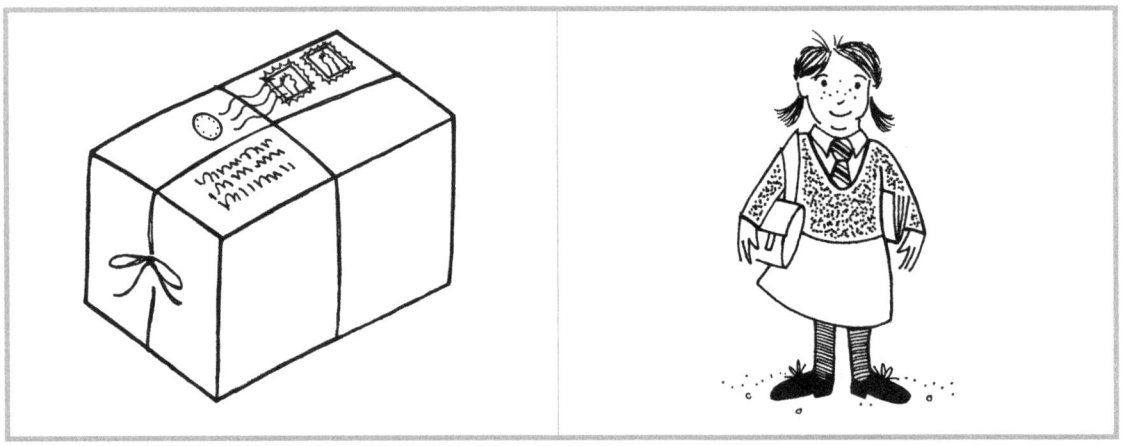

package, pupil

bishop
bigger
busy
budget
bucket
butter
borrow
bother
Bible
basin
beauty
baker
before
begin
beside
behave
behind

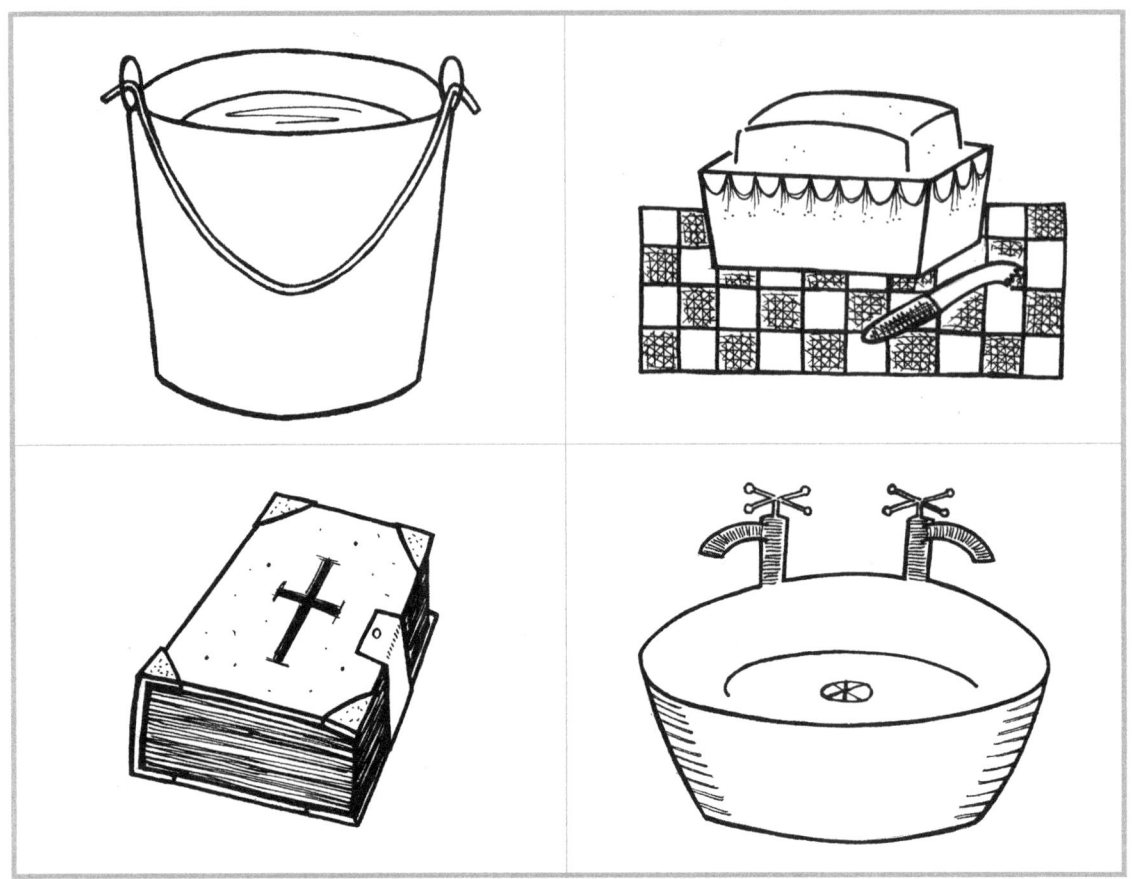

bucket, butter, Bible, basin

Routledge
Taylor & Francis Group

m

menu	major
medal	**mobile**
message	
magic	
manage	
mummy	
moral	

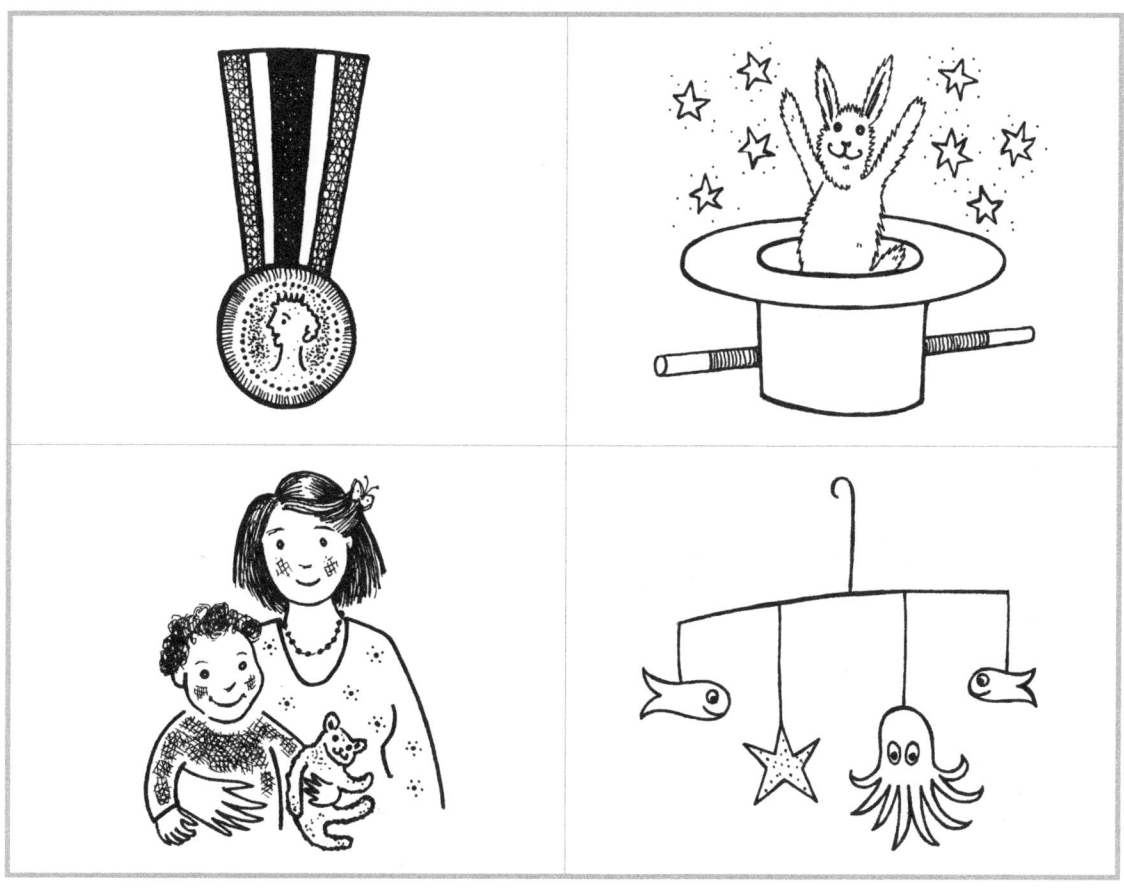

medal, magic, mummy, mobile

209

fishing
finish
figure
finger
filling
follow
forest
fashion
funny
feature
fortune
falling
further
foolish
farmer
famous
faces
favour
forgive

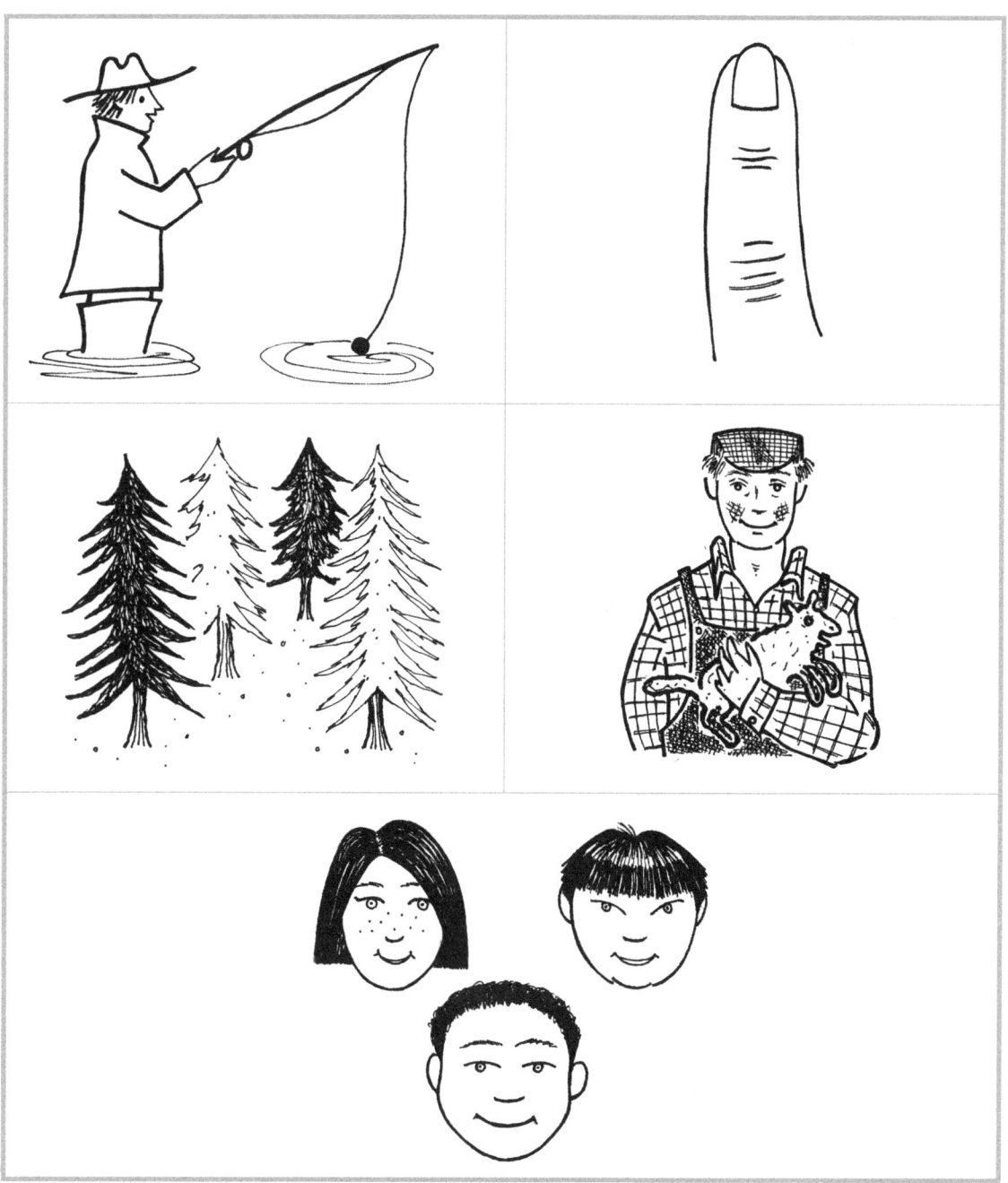

fishing, finger, forest, farmer, faces

visit

villa

victim

value

valid

venue

Venice

verbal

varied

virus

thirty
Thursday
theory
thousand

30	1000

thirty, thousand

th *(as in this)*

thereby
therefore

tissue	timing
topic	title
temper	**tower**
teacher	**toilet**
target	tonight

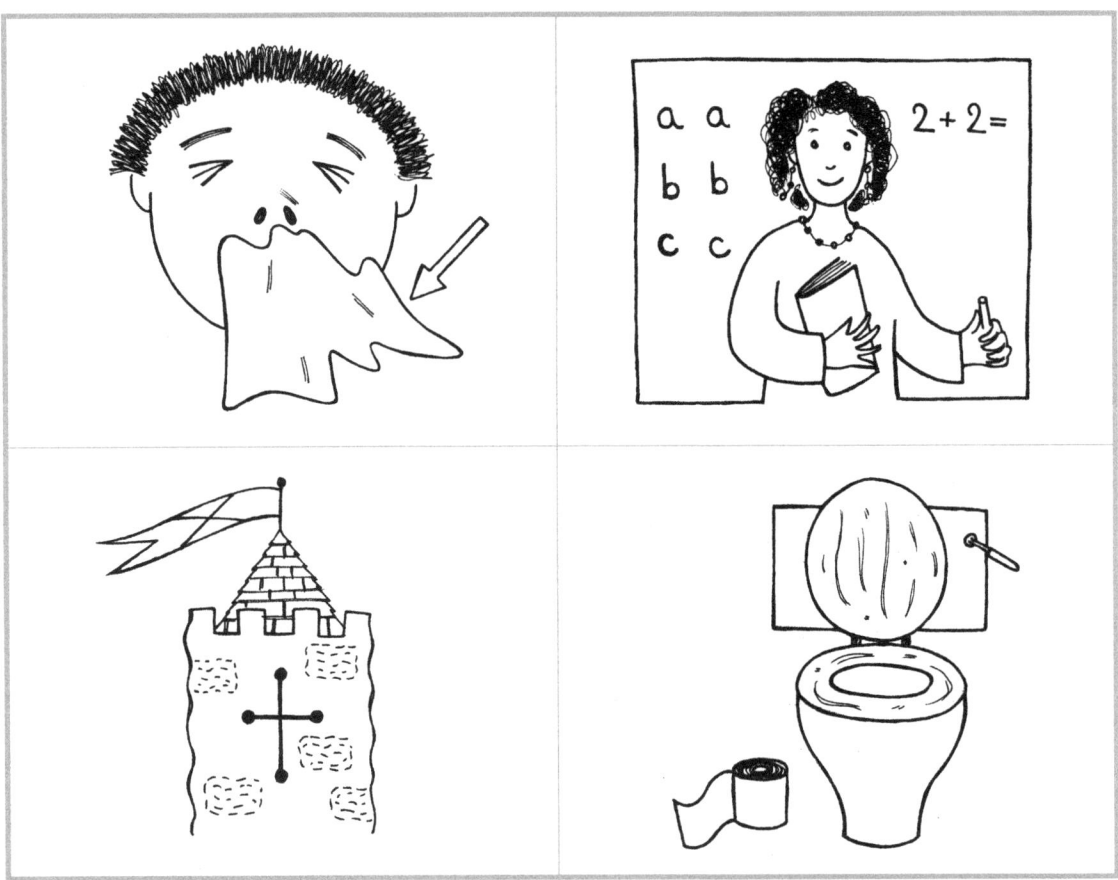

tissue, teacher, tower, toilet

decade
Devon
differ
dishes
damage
daddy
dirty
detail
daughter
depart
debate
design
divide
define
devise

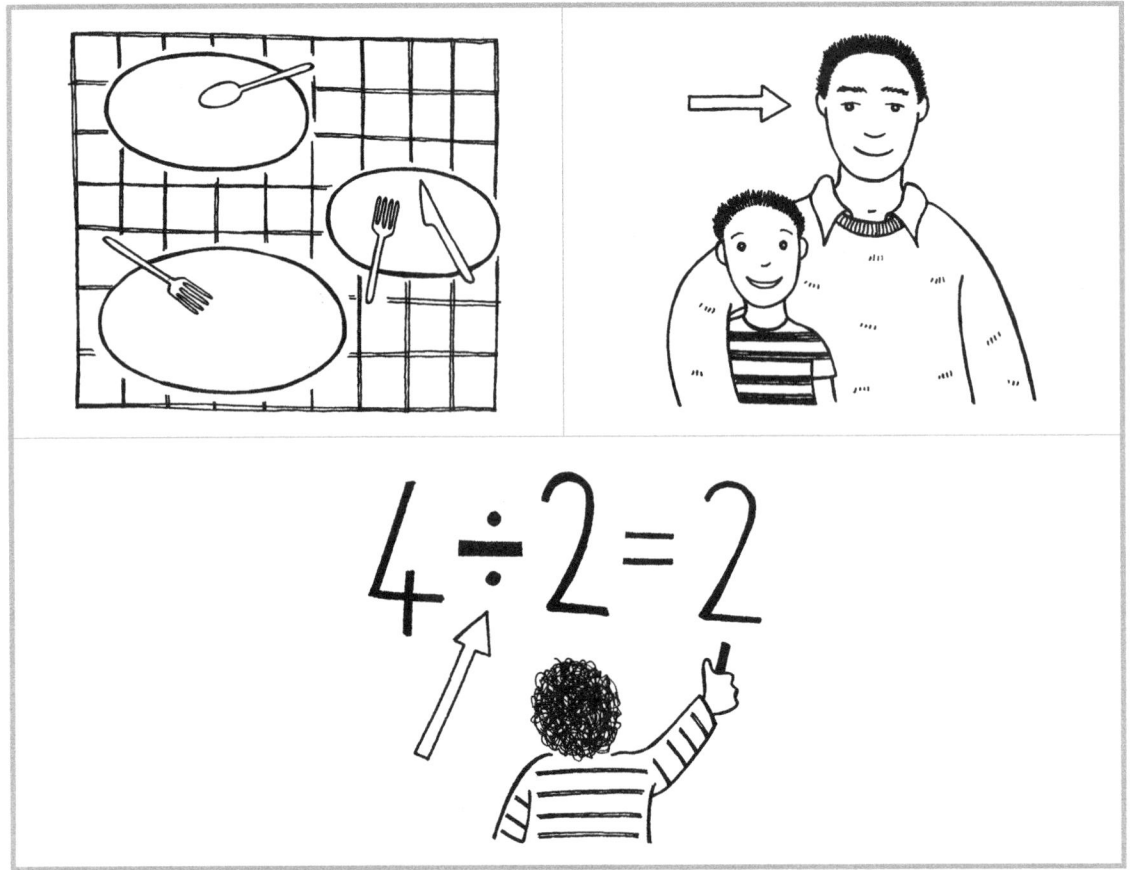

dishes, daddy, divide

network
nothing
needle
navy
nation
nature
knowing
noisy
nightmare

session

singing

sitting

civil

sunny

sudden

supper

suffer

servant

ceiling

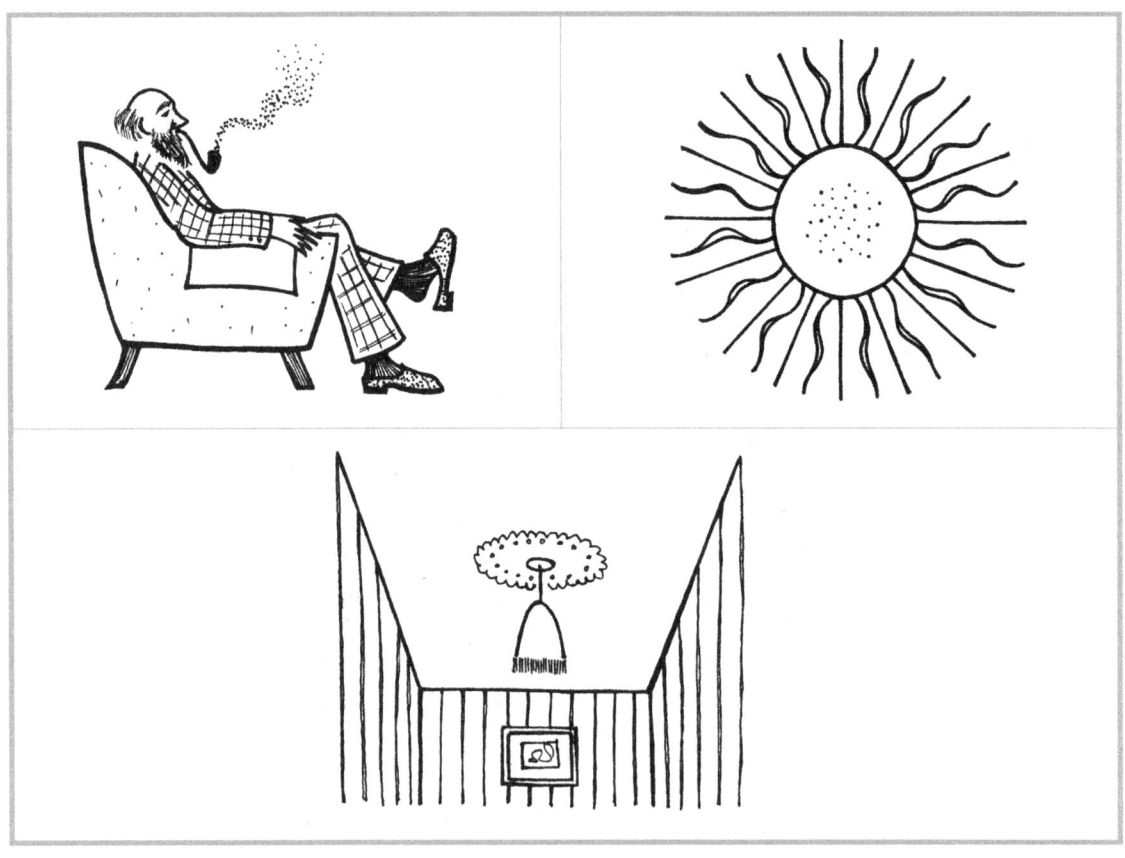

sitting, sunny, ceiling

z

zero

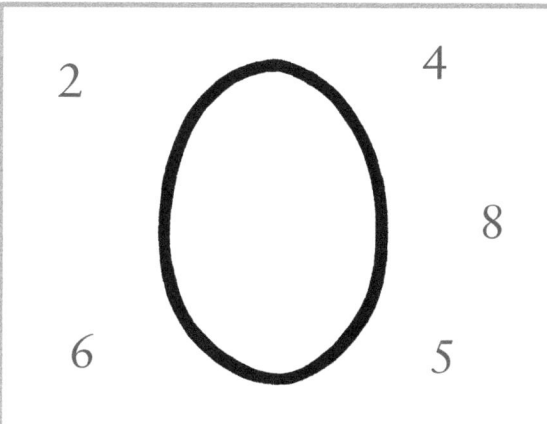

shelter	sharing
shadow	**shoulder**
shopping	**shower**
shooting	showing
shorter	

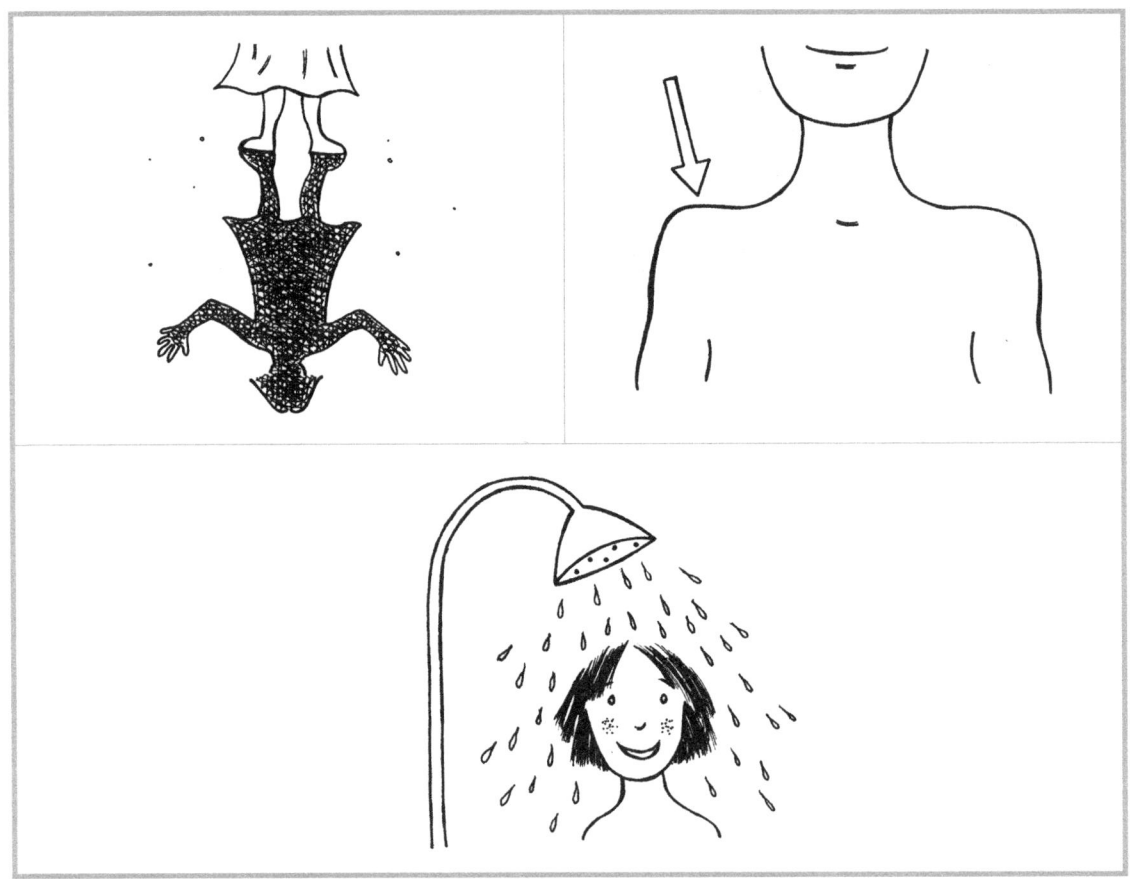

shadow, shoulder, shower

ch

chicken
children
challenge
chapel
channel
chewing
charming
cheerful

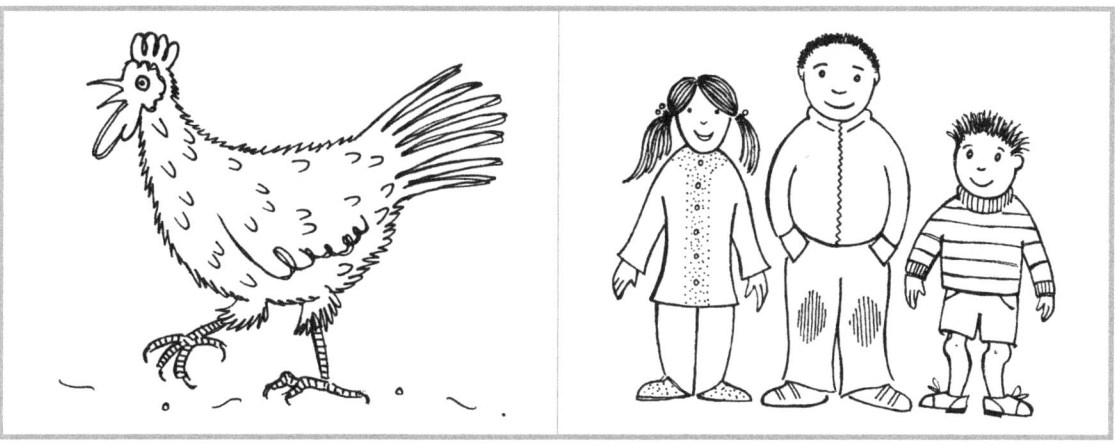

chicken, children

jacket
jungle
judgement
junction
journey
journal
junior
joining
Japan

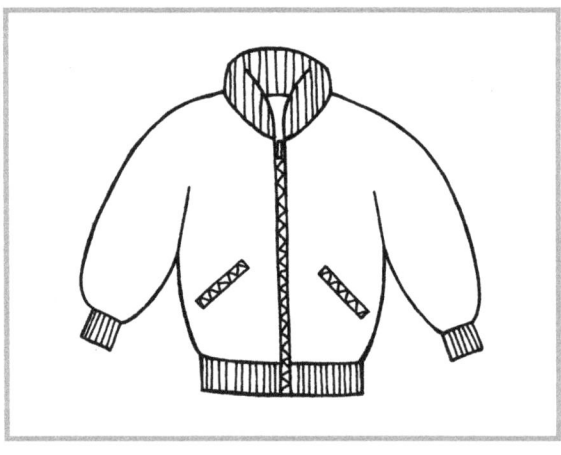

jacket

k

cabin
carriage
copy
common
collar
cutting
colour
current
calling
career

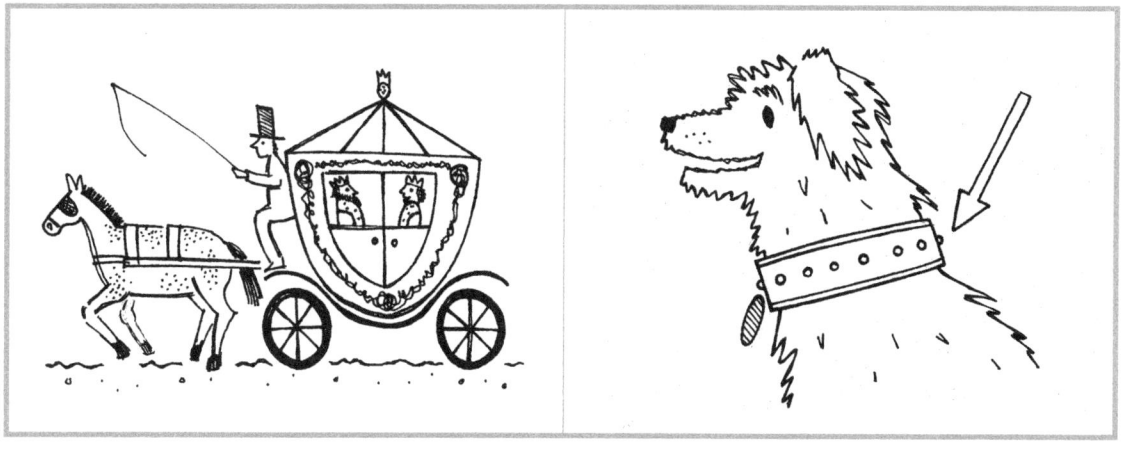

carriage, collar

g

garage
gather
grammar
giving
guilty
gothic
garden
guidance

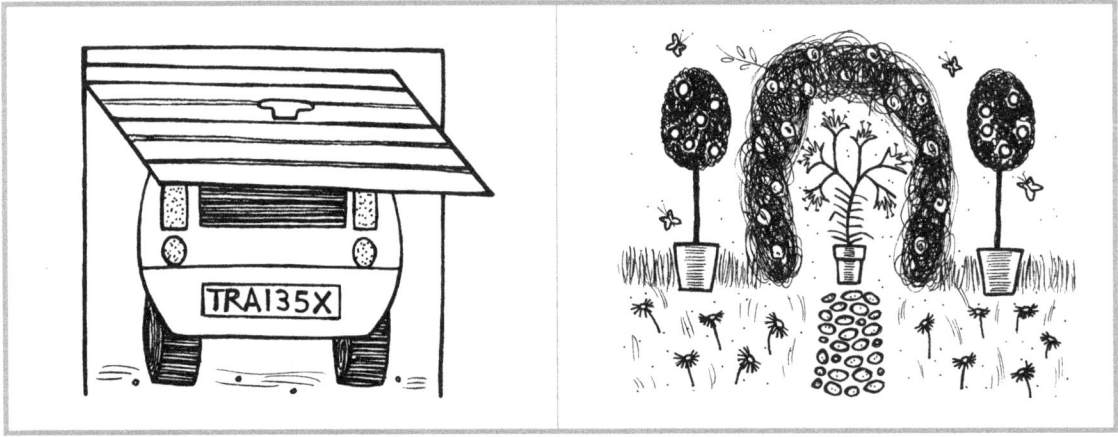

garage, garden

weapon	worthy
wealthy	warning
weather	**wardrobe**
window	**walking**
watching	waiting
woman	

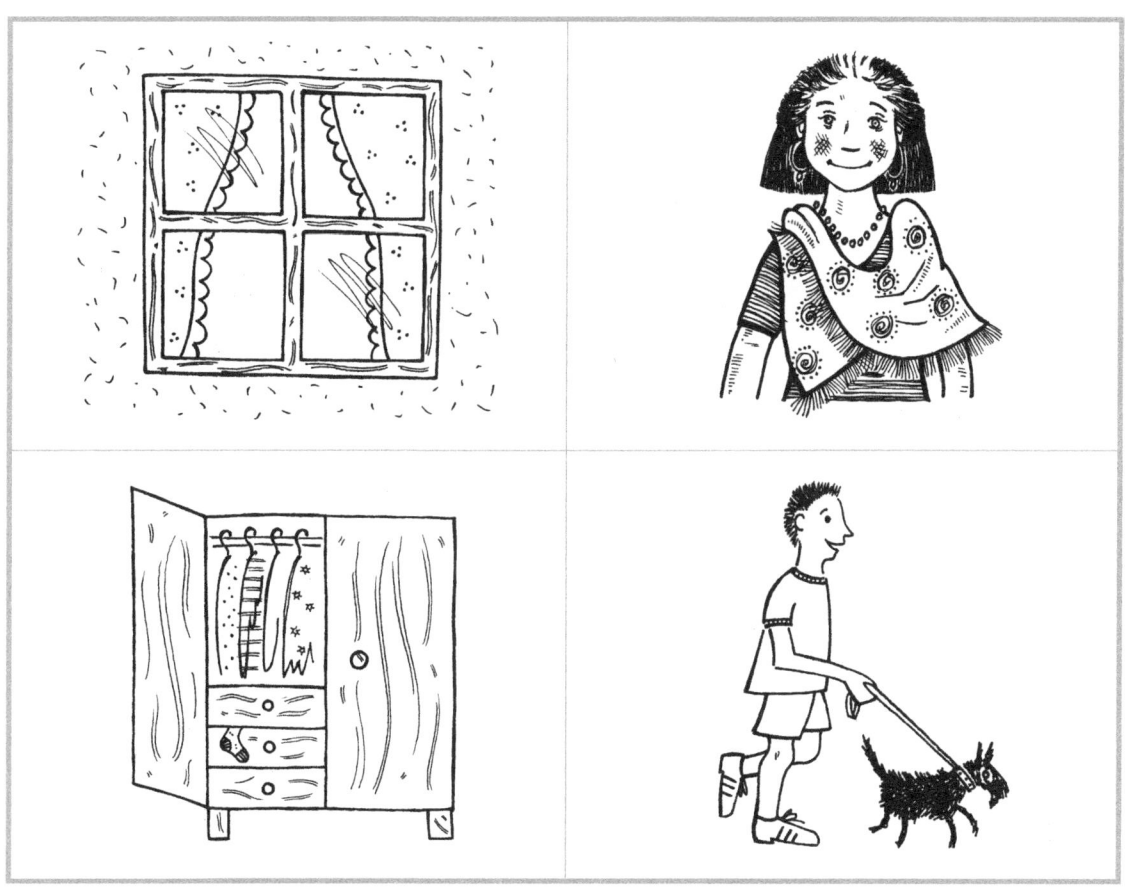

window, woman, wardrobe, walking

r

river
rabbit
robin
rubbish
running
writing
report
reward
refer
repair
resign

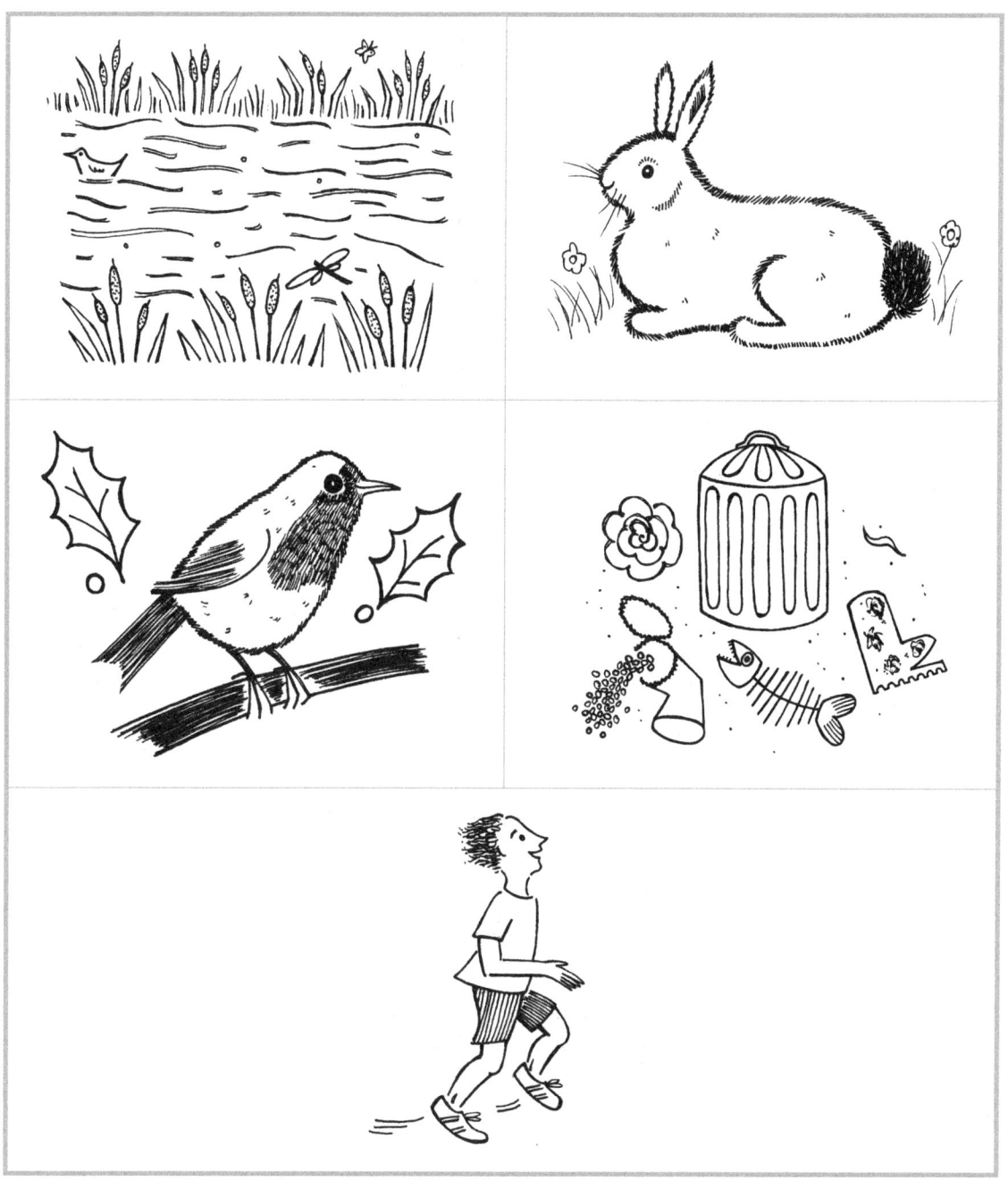

river, rabbit, robin, rubbish, running

l

leather
letter
lesson
lemon
listen
little
logic
lucky
local
loyal

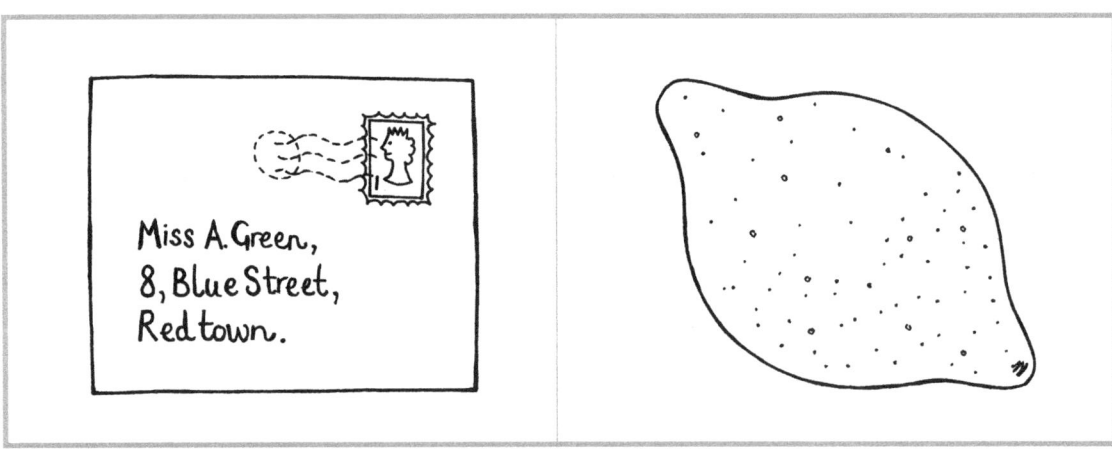

letter, lemon

j

yellow

heaven
heavy
hidden
happy
habit
holly
honey
hungry
husband
human

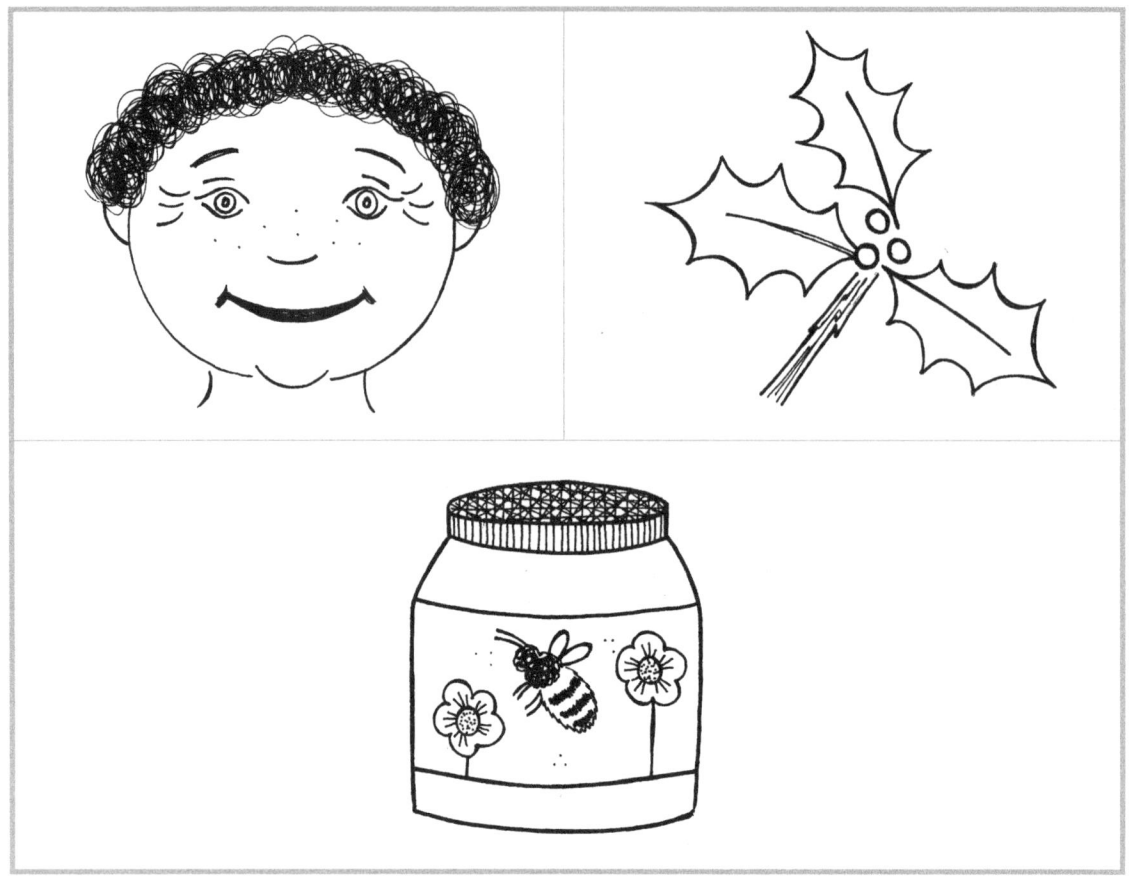

happy, holly, honey

3 or more syllables

p

3 syllables	4 syllables	5 syllables	6 syllables
paragraph	positively	predominantly	
parallel			
passenger	participate	Palestinian	
positive	particular	possibility	
poverty	publicity	probability	
		productivity	
parliament	population	parliamentary	
	publication	popularity	
pacific		personality	
permission			
petition		privatisation	
		participation	
pollution			

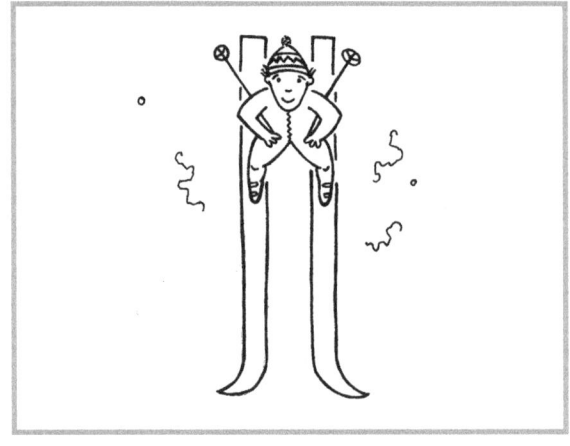

parallel

b

3 syllables	4 syllables	5 syllables	6 syllables
barrier	bureaucracy	biological	
benefit			
burial			
borrowing			
bargaining			
beautiful			
beginning			
belonging			
believing			
behaviour			

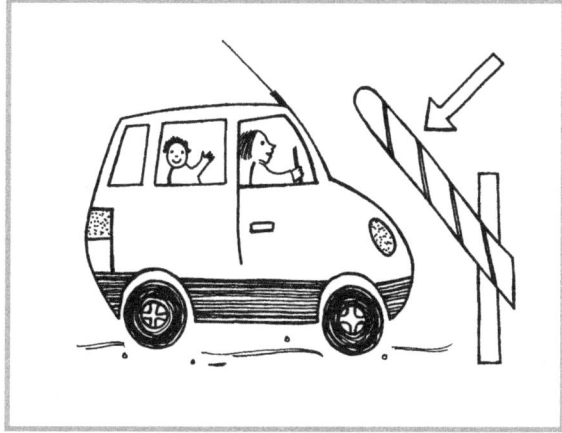

barrier

233

3 syllables	4 syllables	5 syllables	6 syllables
majesty	mortality	manufacturer	
Manchester	morality	manufacturing	
manuscript	mathematical	metropolitan	
mathematics	majority	methodology	
maximum	mobility		
management	maturity	ministerial	
membership	mysterious		
miserable		modification	
military	motivation		
miracle			
monarchy			
maintenance			
motorway			

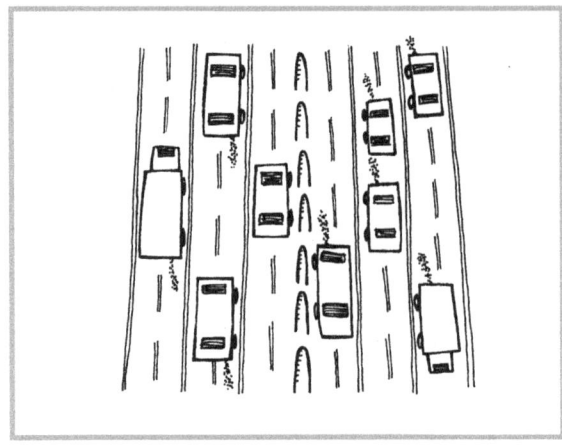

motorway

f

3 syllables	4 syllables	5 syllables	6 syllables
feminist	fortunately	fascinating	
festival			
fashionable	facilitate	philosophical	
		flexibility	
furniture	fundamental		
finally			
furious			
forever			
fantastic			
formation			
frustration			

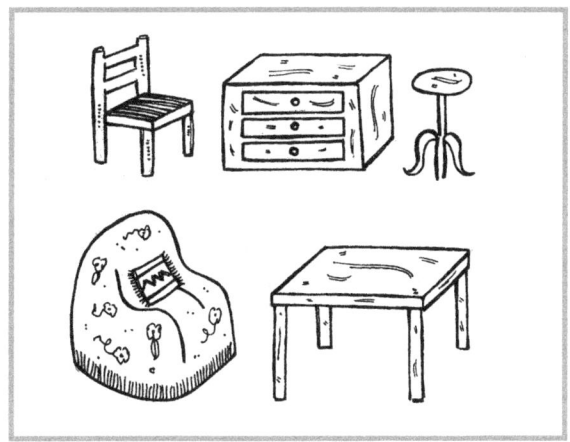

furniture

3 syllables	4 syllables	5 syllables	6 syllables
vegetables	validity	vocabulary	
video	variety		
visible			
visitor	volunteer		
	vegetation		
vertical			

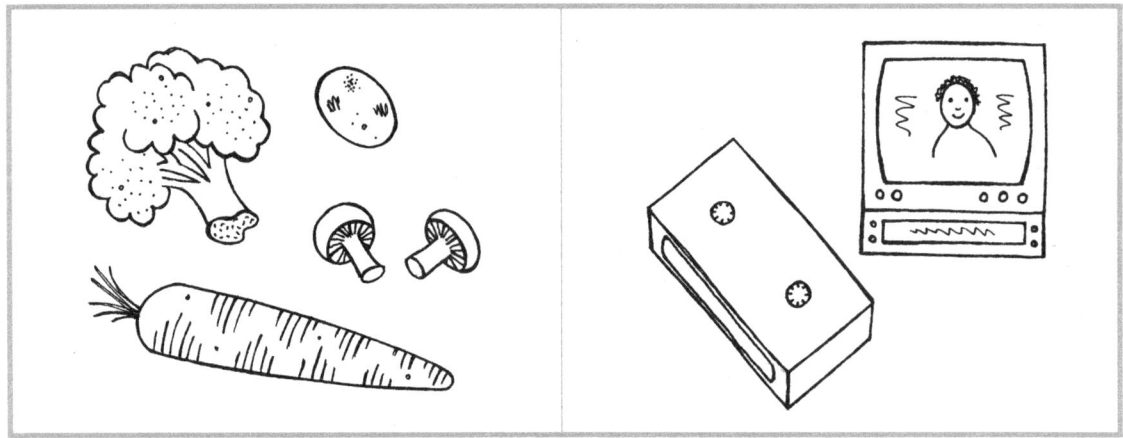

vegetables, video

th *(as in think)*

3 syllables	4 syllables	5 syllables	6 syllables
therapy	theology	theoretical	
threatening			
thoroughly			

3 syllables	4 syllables	5 syllables	6 syllables
technical		technological	
telephone		temporarily	
typical			
		territorial	
tourism			
timetable			
totally			
tobacco			
tomorrow			

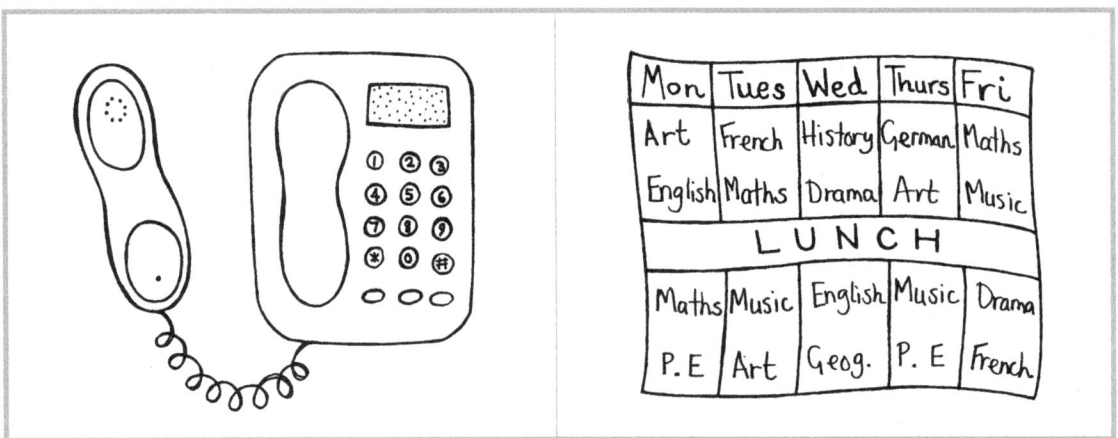

telephone, timetable

d

3 syllables	4 syllables	5 syllables	6 syllables
difficult	development	disciplinary	
database	definition	determination	
dangerous		discrimination	
	diagnosis	documentation	
direction	destination		
December	distribution		
distinction			
division			
disaster			
disorder			
duration			

3 syllables	4 syllables	5 syllables	6 syllables
negative	negotiate	necessarily	
normally		negotiation	
newspaper			
nuclear			
nobody			
November			

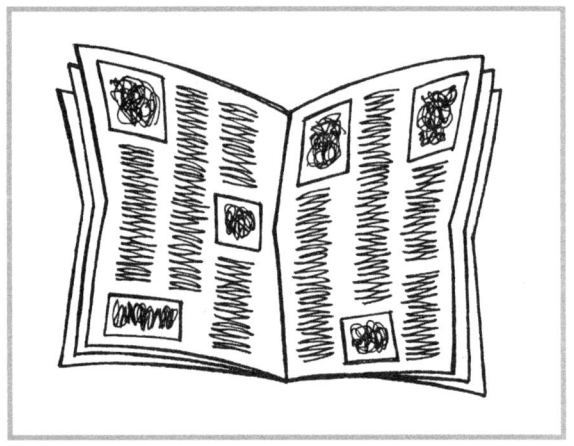

newspaper

3 syllables	4 syllables	5 syllables	6 syllables
salary	**supermarket**	solidarity	simultaneously
satellite		satisfactory	
Saturday	solicitor	significantly	
sensitive	successfully	psychological	
seventy			
signature	security	superintendent	
Switzerland	society	specification	
surgery	satisfaction		
	supervision		
selection	sympathetic		
September			
symbolic	separation		
	situation		
solution			
salvation			

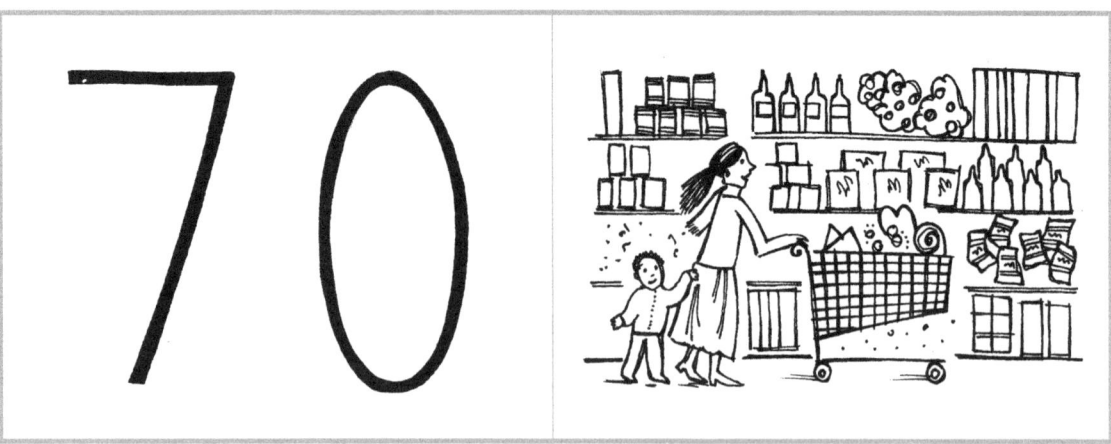

seventy, supermarket

ch

3 syllables	4 syllables	5 syllables	6 syllables
charity			Czechoslovakia
champion			

Although no longer a country, 'Czechoslovakia' provides 6-syllable articulation practice.

j

3 syllables	4 syllables	5 syllables	6 syllables
genuine	generation	geographical	
gentleman		justification	
geography			
January			
justify			
Germany			
journalist			

3 syllables	4 syllables	5 syllables	6 syllables
cabinet	Canadian	capitalism	
calcium	communicate		
calculate	community	constitutional	
calendar			
Canada	competition	characteristic	
capital		Christianity	
caravan	California		
catalogue		classification	
colourful	calculation	cooperation	
countryside	combination	collaboration	
comedy	concentration	communication	
	congregation	configuration	
carefully	conservation	consideration	
	conversation		
collection			
cathedral			
computer			

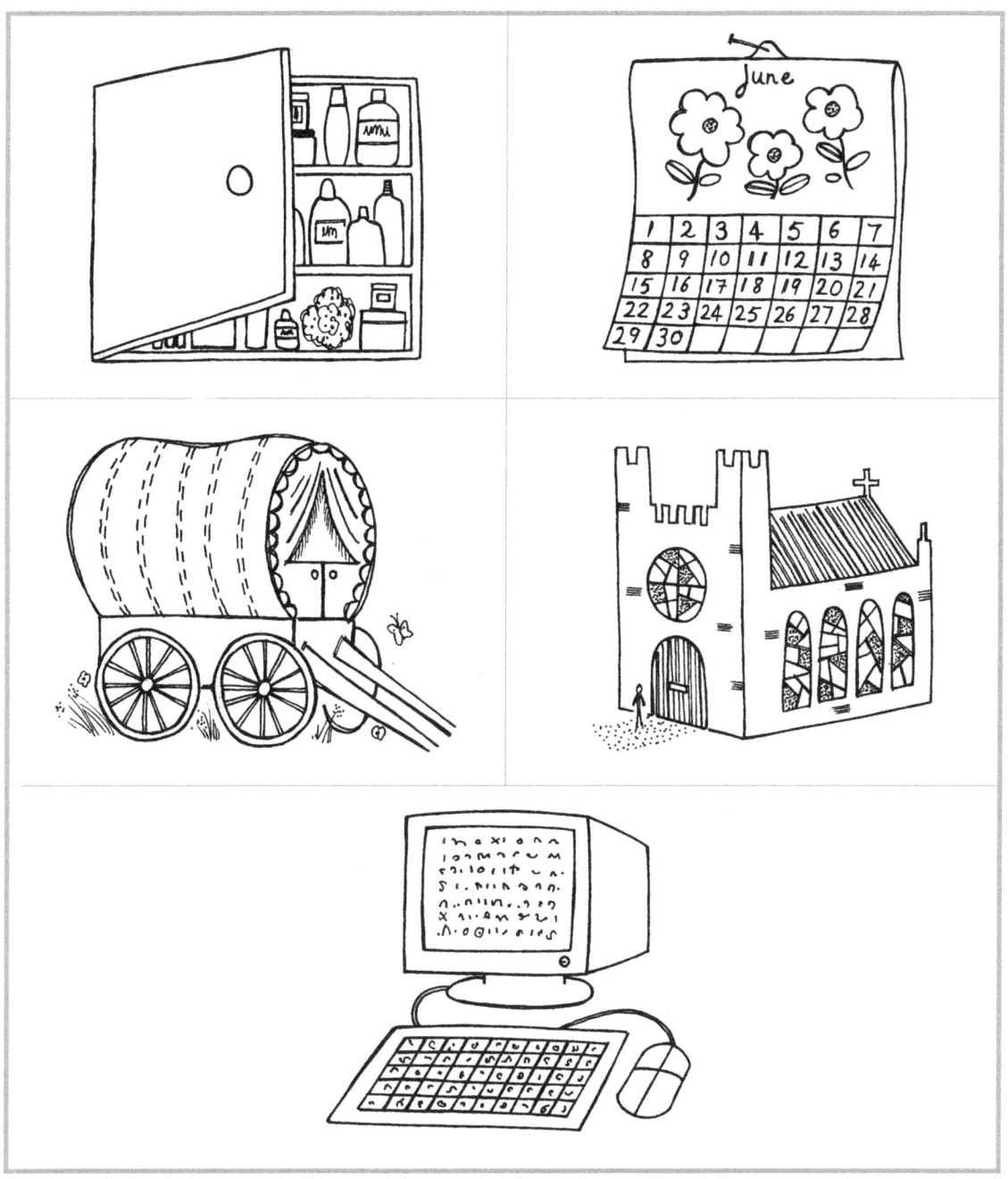

cabinet, calendar, caravan, cathedral, computer

3 syllables	4 syllables	5 syllables	6 syllables
gallery			
governor			
guarantee			

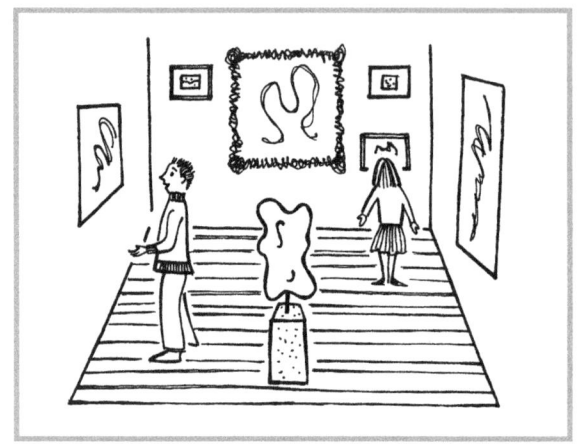

gallery

3 syllables	4 syllables	5 syllables	6 syllables
Washington			
wonderful			
Wimbledon			
worrying			
whatever			

3 syllables	4 syllables	5 syllables	6 syllables
rapidly	reality	representative	
recognise	redundancy		
register	ridiculous	representation	
		recommendation	
reaction	recognition		
romantic	reconstruction		
reception	reproduction		
reflection			
redundant	radiation		
	registration		
reporter	reputation		
removal			
reminder			
refugee			

l

3 syllables	4 syllables	5 syllables	6 syllables
Lancashire	laboratory	liability	
liberty	legitimate		
literature			
Liverpool	liberation		
logical	legislation		
leadership			
loyalty			
location			

y

3 syllables	4 syllables	5 syllables	6 syllables
yesterday			

3 syllables	4 syllables	5 syllables	6 syllables
habitat	hostility		
handicap	humanity		
happiness			
holiday			
horrible			
hospital			
harmony			
headmaster			
horizon			

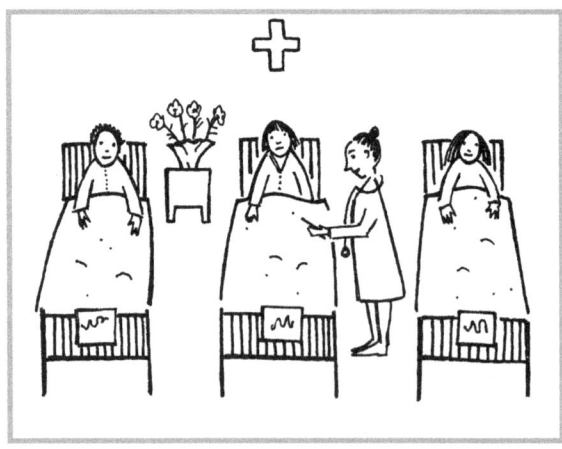

hospital

LEMON & LIME LIBRARY OF PHRASES & SENTENCES

5

The phrases and sentences of the Lemon & Lime library are available from this chapter or from the CD-Rom where they can be accessed under Level 7.

The phrases are organised according to the target phoneme as for the short and multisyllabic words in part 2 of the resource pack. There are two pages related to each consonant sound. The first of these presents three lists of short phrases, which contain only one word with the target phoneme. The phoneme precedes short and long vowels and diphthongs. The second page presents two lists of sound saturated sentences, or tongue twisters, the first list containing shorter phrases and sentences, and the second containing yet more challenging, longer sentences.

After each sound has been presented as the sole target at sentence level, this chapter is completed by presenting phrases and sentences for practising more than one placement, or manner of articulation. This can be used for a varied practice schedule as motor learning theory recommends, helping the process of generalisation of learned sounds into spontaneous speech. It can also be used as a means to practise producing distinct minimally contrasting sounds in connected speech: for example 'she sells sea shells on the sea shore', as opposed to 'see sells sea sells on the see saw' or 'she shells she shells on the she shore'.

Phrases & sentences targeting bilabials

Phrases & sentences targeting labiodentals

Phrases & sentences targeting inter-dentals

Phrases & sentences targeting alveolar stops & nasals

Phrases & sentences targeting alveolar & post alveolar fricatives

Phrases & sentences targeting affricates

Phrases & sentences targeting velar stops

Phrases & sentences targeting approximants

With short vowels

I write with a **pen**

My vegetable **patch**

An orange **pip**

The balloon went **pop**

My dog is a **pup**

Pull and **push**

With long vowels

War and **peace**

A string of **pearls**

Play in the **park**

Roast pork

The front **porch**

With diphthongs

You have to **pay**

Apple **pie**

What is your **point**?

A game of **poker**

Fifty **pounds**

Orange **peel**

Juicy **pear**

Phrases

Picking apple pips

Pork pies for a picnic

Put pen to paper

Pass the popcorn please

Pay Polly for the pie

Poor Peter's poorly

Sentences

The poor pirate paid for his peppers with peas

Pick Paul up from the porch at Polly's please

Pippa pored over pages and pages of the play

Peter and Paul picked pounds of peaches to put in their pockets

Poppy pushed the pink pig in the park

b – target consonant in one word

With short vowels

A rubbish **bin**

Go to **bed**

A cricket **bat**

Robert or **Bob**

A red **bus**

Read a good **book**

With long vowels

I was stung by a **bee**

New Wellington **boots**

That dog will **bark**

Where were you **born?**

When is your **birthday?**

With diphthongs

A little **baby**

Ride a motor **bike**

Put the kettle on to **boil**

A fishing **boat**

A cool **beer**

Teddy **bear**

b – saturated phrases and sentences

Phrase/short sentences

Big bouncing baby

Buy bread and butter

The book bored Bob

Bill bought a badge

Baker's bread is best

Bring Ben a beer

Beaten black and blue

Sentences

Bill asked Ben if he was born in a barn

Bad Barney barked and barked for butcher's beef

Bobby Brown broke Barry's bike

Can Barry bake buns to take on the boat?

The bath water was black after Barney's bath

Bill and Ben were born in Burgh on Bain

Ben bought bluebells for Betty's birthday

m – target consonant in one word

Words with short vowels

A flour **mill**

What a **mess**

You need a **map**

A floor **mop**

A cup or a **mug?**

Words with long vowels

Cheese or **meat?**

A full **moon**

Ask for **mercy**

Make your **mark**

I want **more**

Words with diphthongs

What did you **make?**

That's **mine**

Don't **moan**

Open your **mouth**

A delicious **meal**

He ran a **mile**

Short phrases / sentences

Mark's mean with his money

I miss Molly on Mondays

More meat for the meal

My modern map

Mum missed the match

Mike's mum is mean

Sentences

Mick and Mandy had a meal at the mill

Mark's in a mean mood on Monday morning

Where's my modern map of Manchester?

May needs much more meat for Muppet's meals

My main mission is to make much more money

Miss Mop meets Mickey Mouse a mile from Mark's mum's mansion

Paul bought me a pint of beer

Bobby paid for my trip to Bombay

May brought me a piece of maple syrup pie

Peter blamed me for making a big mess

There was a mouse peeping at me from behind the paper mill

Mushy peas, pie and chips is a most welcome meal when I'm in a bad mood

The man in the moon is a comfort to most people when they are in bed

More money doesn't bring many people peace

Poppies, bluebells and marigolds make me happy

Make your mark by helping the poor

f – target consonant in one word

Words with short vowels

Does it **fit?**

She **fell**

Turn on the **fan**

It's **full**

Words with long vowels

You've got big **feet?**

Enjoy your **food**

I came **first**

Where's the **farm?**

That car is a **Ford**

Words with diphthongs

A summer **fête**

The weather is **fine**

Is it your **phone?**

Look what I've **found!**

That's my biggest **fear**

It's not **fair**

f – saturated phrases and sentences

Short phrases/sentences

Four fine flowers

Five funny fingers

Felicity flew to Florida

Florence found a fortune

Flash floods in the Fens

Only fools fight with foxes

Sentences

Felicity has been friends with Florence for fifty-five years

Frank forgot to find Fay's phone in February

Flo and Frances bought flip-flops for Felicity to take to Florida

Fine food cost Frank and Fay a fortune in France

Flora found five fingers of fudge for her friends in Filey

Fat Fred pulled funny faces at his foolish football fans

Words with short vowels

Where's **Victor**?

Go to the **vets**

My new **van**

Words with long vowels

Read me a **verse**

A flower **vase**

Words with diphthongs

Don't be so **vain**

Grape **vine**

Short phrases/sentences

Victor visited Vicky

Violets in a vase

The vet's van

Victor's vicious viper

Violent Vinny's vain

Longer sentences

Violent Vinny read Vicky a verse

Victor's vet's van is vicious

Vain Vicky voted for Violent Vinny

Vinny and Victor played volley-ball in the vines

Vincent visited Vicky with a vase of violets

Mixed labiodental saturated sentences

Violent Vinny fought for Vicky's fine vase of violets

Vain Vicky pulled funny faces on the phone

Foolish Flora fled from Victor's vicious viper

Vinny found Victor's vet's van far from Vicky's farm

Fresh violets and freesias are my favourite flowers

Flo and Vicky voted to fly to Florida

Words with short vowels

What do you **think**?

Is that a **threat**?

Many **thanks**

Words with long vowels

One two **three**

Come **through**

They came **third**

It's a **thorn**

Words with diphthongs

Look at my **thigh**!

I've got a sore **throat**

Let's go to the **theatre**

Short phrase/sentences

I'm thirty-three on the third

Through thick and thin

Thea threw the thorn

Longer sentences

Thea threatened to go through the theatre

Theo got three thorns in his thick thigh

Thanks to Thea all three went to the theatre on Thursday

Words with short vowels

What's **this**?

What's **that**?

That was **then**

Words with diphthongs

Who are **they**?

Not **those**!

Over **there**

This is one of those days

Let's get those over there with this

That's where they were then!

Those that did this are over there

They couldn't do that therefore they did this

Words with short vowels

The biscuits are in the **tin**

Six seven eight nine **ten**

Turn off the **tap**

Right at the **top**

It weighs a **tonne**

Words with long vowels

A nice cup of **tea**

Is there enough for **two?**

When is it my **turn?**

The road is covered in wet **tar**

The dress is completely **torn**

Words with diphthongs

Her eyes filled with **tears**

Give me the video **tape**

He's not my **type**

I've got a new **toy**

Build a big **tower**

t – saturated phrases and sentences

Short phrases/sentences

Ten tiny toes

Tell me the time

Take me to the toilet

Tony toasted the team

Turn off the tap for the tenth time!

Longer sentences

Can you take me to tea at Tom's on Tuesday?

Try to take time to tune the trumpet tonight

The train to Totnes leaves at two twenty from platform two

Tibby the tiny tabby tipped tea on Tom's trousers

Times of terror on telly turn Tim to tears

d – target consonant in one word

Words with short vowels

There's my **dad**

Put it in a **dish**

She's a bit **deaf**

The ship's in **dock**

Feed the **ducks**

Words with long vowels

The river is very **deep**

Many people are scared of the **dark**

The dog was covered in **dirt**

The birds start to sing at **dawn**

Words with diphthongs

What's the **date?**

I was left in no **doubt**

272

Short phrases/sentences

The dog dived for the duck

Dating Dave is dangerous

Don't do dishes in the dark

Daniel's dad is deaf

Don drives from dawn til dusk

Longer sentences

Don't you dare deafen Dave with the drums

Don doesn't drive down to Devon dangerously

Daniel reached his distinctive destination of Dubai by December

Does Dave's dog have a diagnosed disorder?

I dreamed it was difficult to dive in the dark when drunk

Words with short vowels

You're a pain in the **neck**

No it's **not!**

Would you like a **nut?**

I can **knit**

Words with long vowels

I've hurt my **knee**

It's cold in the **north**

My daughter is a **nurse**

Words with diphthongs

What's your **name?**

That's **nice**

He left a **note**

Don't be so **noisy!**

Short phrases/sentences

It's a nice night Nick

Nobody knows Nanny

The nurse's name is Nora

There's nothing new to know

A nice navy nightdress

Longer sentences

There's no need to know how to knit nowadays

Naughty Nina knows not to knock on doors in the night

The note named Nora the nurse as the one who knew

Nora never needed knitted wear in November

It's nice to know the people in the north are nice

Tom and Dina had dinner tonight with nine men from the navy

Dan and Nina don't drink tea in tents

Tony drove to Devon at ninety from north Tyneside

Nobody knew Dianne turned Tony into a terrific drummer

Nina's dog terrified ten tiny ducks today for nothing

Dan's nanny was nicknamed Dot the dangerous when she drove Dina to tears after drinking gin

Words with short vowels

The TV **set**

She looks **sad**

Where's my **sock**?

A bright yellow **sun**

The postman's **sack**

Words with long vowels

Can I have **soup**?

Where's my **seat**?

Tomato **sauce**

Words with diphthongs

Don't worry, you're **safe**

Which **side**?

Wash with **soap**

The envelope **seal**

s – saturated phrases and sentences

Short phrases/sentences

Sixty-seven soldiers

Sow seeds in the sun

Salmon sandwiches are special

Simon's smelly sock

Such sorrow is sad

Longer sentences

Sixty-seven silky soapsuds sparkling for us to see

Seven silly sisters sat sipping sangria on the soft sofa

Say sorry to Sarah for stealing her son's socks

Simon and Sarah were so sad to see their son go to sea

The sea seems silver at sunset

Words with short vowels

I broke the **zip**

From A to **Z**

Words with long vowels

Let's go to the **zoo**

Words with diphthongs

The red **zone**

z – saturated phrases and sentences

Short phrases/sentences

Zebras at the zoo

Zippy's in the red zone

Longer sentences

There were zero zebras in the blue zone of the zoo

Words with short vowels

I can see a **ship!**

The garden **shed**

Can you go to the **shop?**

The door is **shut**

Words with long vowels

My hair is **short**

Hands up or I'll **shoot!**

Iron my **shirt**

Counting **sheep**

The knife is **sharp**

Words with diphthongs

Put the baby in the **shade**

It's nice to **share**

Don't **shout**

The sun **shines**

Short phrases sentences

The shop is shut

Shall we shear the sheep?

Sheryl went shopping with Shona

Sheryl's shoes are shiny

The ship shone as it came ashore

Longer sentences

Sheryl shopped with Shona for shoes, shampoo and a shirt

The bishop showed the nation that he could shout

Shelly paid cash for a portion of fish on the shore

The sheriff showed Sheryl that he could shear sheep in the shed

She sells sea shells on the sea shore

Simon sold Sheryl a short sleeved shirt and shiny silver shoes

She was sure it was Simon who stole sweets from the shop

The shiny ship sailed on the still ocean

Sally shut the shop for the show on Saturday

The shop at the zoo sold soft zebras, special sweets and stuffed sheep

Words with short vowels

A jolly good **chap**

A pork **chop**

Did you **check**?

Take it on the **chin**

Words with long vowels

It's really **cheap**

Where's the **chart**?

You can **choose**

Words with diphthongs

Look at that **chain**!

What a **choice**!

They let out a **cheer**

Short phrases/sentences

Charlie wore checked chinos

The chap chewed the chop

Choose chips and cheese

Choose cheap cheese

They cheered when the chick cheeped

Longer sentences

Chips and cheese are much cheaper in March

Teach the children to chop cheese in the kitchen

Words with short vowels

Strawberry **jam**

Do you like **jazz?**

Let's go by **jet**

That's your **job!**

Words with long vowels

It's in the **jar**

An aching **jaw**

Orange **juice**

Words with diphthongs

The burglar is in **jail**

Do you want to **join?**

Is that a **joke?**

Short phrases/sentences

It's a large jam jar

Gerry joked with John

The joy rider joined Joe in jail

Jane jumped over the hedge

John's orange was juicy

Longer sentences

Jane jilted Gerry at St John's in July

The judge put John in jail from January to July

k – target in one word

Words with short vowels

Give me a **kiss**

Can you **come?**

Get a **cab**

Words with long vowels

Keep **calm**

Open the **curtains**

Get in the **car**

Words with diphthongs

A piece of **cake**

A dark **cave**

The fire needs more **coal**

Where's my **coat?**

She gave me a **coin**

k – saturated phrases and sentences

Short phrases/sentences

Can you come to Colin's?

Kate's Christmas cake

Take care in the cave

Chris cleaned the car

Claire's colourful coat

Longer sentences

Can Colin and Kate come to the caravan in Cork?

The king of the castle likes coming to the common in his carriage

Claire and Keith count caravans to keep them occupied in the car

Kate came across a colourful coin in her cardigan pocket

Colin tried to keep the kids calm in the car crash

Words with short vowels

I can smell **gas**

Mind the **gap**

That's **good**

Do you believe in **God**?

What can you **give**?

Words with long vowels

It's a **girl!**

The changing of the **guards**

Words with diphthongs

Open the **gate**

He's a nice **guy**

He scored a **goal**

Change **gear**

Are you ready to **go**?

g – saturated phrases and sentences

Short phrases/sentences

Go and get Gordon

Give granny a gift

Guss was a good guy

Gaynor is a girl guide

Grandad's got geese in the garden

Longer sentences

The Girl Guides giggled at the gift they gave Gordon

Go and get Gaynor from Granny's garden

Grandad is going to give Gordon an organ when he is bigger

Granny keeps goats, geese, pigs and an eagle in her garden

Guy forgave Glenn for getting the goal

Can Gordon go to Gaynor's Granny's for Christmas?

Grandad's car can go fast when he gets the correct gear

Catherine can go to Kenya again with Kate at Christmas

Could Connor give Gary his computer game to keep him occupied?

Going to Guides can give girls confidence

Gaynor can keep Granny's geese comfortable when the climate gets cold

Words with short vowels

Who **with?**

You're all **wet!**

So **what!**

Who **would!**

Words with long vowels

See you next **week**

Spread the **word**

Shall we go for a **walk?**

Words with diphthongs

What do you **weigh?**

I don't know **why**

That's **weird!**

I don't know what to **wear**

Short phrases/sentences

Where's Wendy's wand?

What did you wish for?

Walter walked to Wales!

Longer sentences

Willow the Wisp waited for the wicked witch

Why is the weather wet on Wednesdays?

Walter walked for weeks and weeks until he was worn out

Words with short vowels

Give me a **ring**

I like **red**

I saw a **rat!**

You're **wrong!**

Words with long vowels

A book to **read**

Don't be **rude**

The lion **roared**

Words with diphthongs

She won the **race**

I think you're **right**

Cross the **road**

They had a **row**

r – saturated phrases and sentences

Short phrases/sentences

A single red rose

Have you seen my Rolls-Royce?

Ryan reads rubbish

Ryan gave Rose a ruby ring

Longer sentences

Richard and Ryan rowed rapidly down the River Rase

Robert knows the right road to Rochdale

Richard is rarely rude to Rose when she is wrong

A row of roses grows round Robert and Rachel's red front door

Words with short vowels

As heavy as **lead**

I remember when I was a **lad**

Keep the door **locked**

She's in **love**

Words with long vowels

The roof **leaks**

Her tooth is **loose**

You've got to **learn!**

A lump of **lard**

Words with diphthongs

You're **late!**

Do what you **like**

It's hard to bear the **load**

The music is too **loud**

l – saturated phrases and sentences

Short phrases/sentences

Lucy likes lemons

Load the leaves onto the lorry

Leon loves Lisa

Larry climbed the ladder

Longer sentences

Lucy lay in the lounge licking her lemon lolly

Larry lent Leon his ladder to load the lorry

Leaves are a lot lighter to load on the lorry than lumps of lead

Larry was leaping like a lion because he was livid that the music was too loud

Words with short vowels

Not **yet!**

Have you seen my **yacht?**

She's so **young**

Words with long vowels

Where are **you?**

In the **yard**

I need to **yawn**

Words with diphthongs

In which **year?**

y – saturated phrases and sentences

Short phrases/sentences

Where's your yo-yo?

You're still young yet

Longer sentences

Can we use your yellow yacht this year?

You're too young to drive a Yaris yet

Words with short vowels

I need my **hat**

I've got a bald **head**

Walk up the **hill**

It's too **hot**

Words with long vowels

The compost **heap**

Jump through the **hoop**

She's got a good **heart**

Beep the **horn**

Words with diphthongs

A bail of **hay**

Put it up **high**

Don't give up **hope**

I can't **hear**

Short phrases/sentences

How high Harry?

Have you had a hot dog?

Hilda had a heavy heart

How is Horace's horse?

Longer sentences

Harry had a hat to help keep the hot sun off his head

Harry helped Horace heap hay for the horse

Henry has high hopes for his holiday in Hawaii

REFERENCES

Ball M, Rahilly J & Tench P, 1996, *The Phonetic Transcription of Disordered Speech*, Singular Publishing Group, London.

Dean E, Howell J, Hill A & Waters D, 1991, *The Metaphon Resource Pack*, NFER-Nelson, Windsor.

Fletcher SG, 1992, *Articulation: A Physiological Approach*, Singular Publishing Group, San Diego, p213.

Gimson A, 1980, *An Introduction to the Pronunciation of English*, Edward Arnold, London.

Grunwell P, 1992, *Clinical Phonology*, 2nd edn, Chapman and Hall, London.

Howell J & Dean E, 1991, *Treating Phonological Disorders in Children: Metaphon – Theory to Practice*, Whurr, London.

Kay J, Lesser R & Coltheart M, 1992, *PALPA: Psycholinguistic Assessment of Language Processing in Aphasia*, Lawrence Erlbaum, Hove.

Lange C, Unnithan V, Larkam E & Latta P, 2000, Maximising the Benefits of Pilates-Inspired Exercise for Learning Functional Motor Skills, *Journal of Bodywork and Movement Therapies*, 4 (2), pp99–108.

Leech G, Rayson P & Wilson A, 2001, *Word Frequencies in Written and Spoken English based on the British National Corpus*, Pearson, Harlow.

Palmer C & Meyer RK, 2000, Conceptual and Motor Learning in Music Performance, *Psychological Science*, 11 (1), pp63–68.

Swigert NB, 1997, *The Source for Dysarthria*, Linguisystems, East Moline.

Wulf G & Schmidt R, 1997, Variability of Practice and Implicit Motor Learning, *Journal of Experimental Psychology: Learning, Memory and Cognition*, 23 (4), pp63–68.

Yorkston KM, Beukelman DR, Strand EA & Bell KR, 1999, *Management of Motor Speech Disorders in Children and Adults*, 2nd edn, Pro-Ed, Texas.